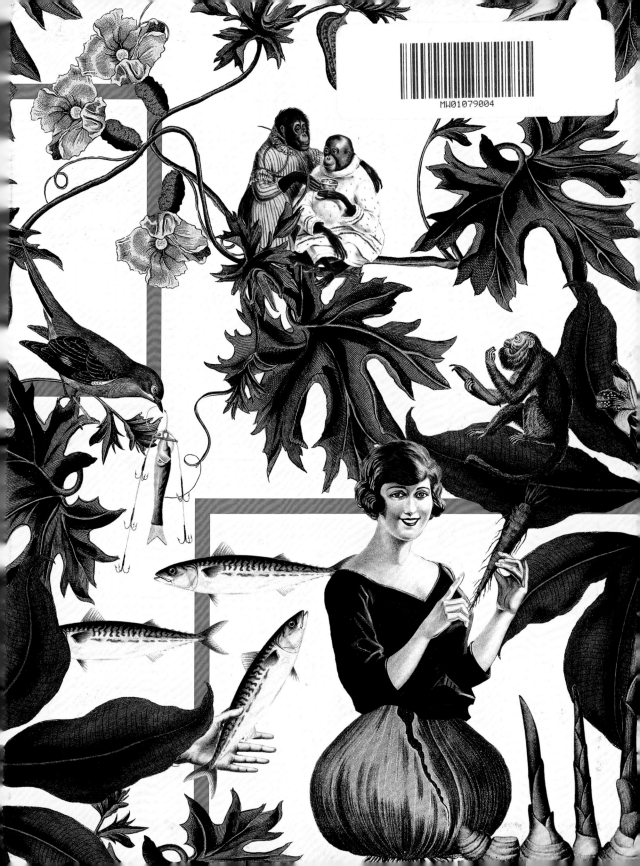

MW01079004

FOOD PI+\RMACY

**A Guide to Gut Bacteria,
Anti-Inflammatory Foods, and
Eating for Health**

**A prescription diet you will never
overdose on.**

*Lina Nertby Aurell & Mia Clase
Translation by Gun Penhoat*

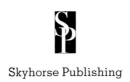

Skyhorse Publishing

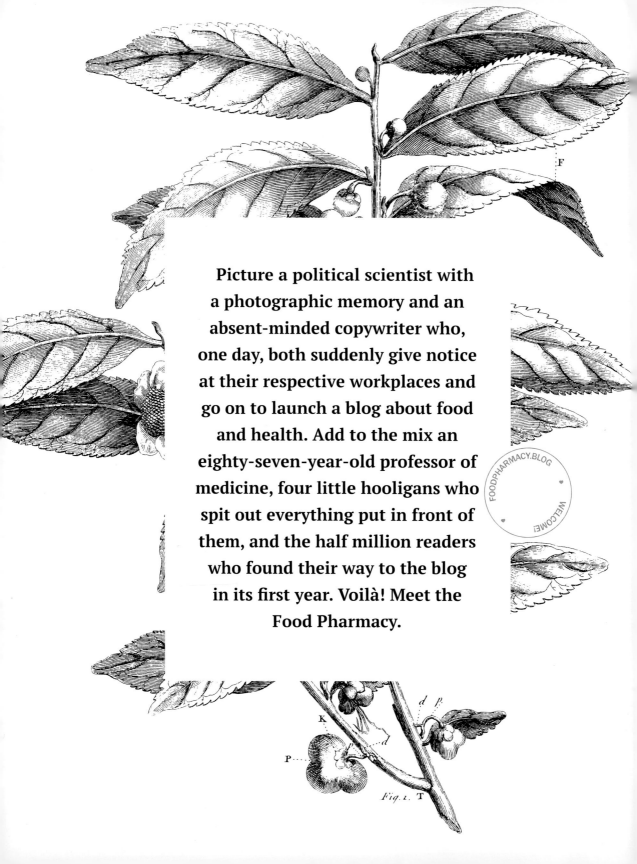

Picture a political scientist with a photographic memory and an absent-minded copywriter who, one day, both suddenly give notice at their respective workplaces and go on to launch a blog about food and health. Add to the mix an eighty-seven-year-old professor of medicine, four little hooligans who spit out everything put in front of them, and the half million readers who found their way to the blog in its first year. Voilà! Meet the Food Pharmacy.

CONTENTS

SCIENCE FOR YOU

Page

WE ARE LINA AND MIA. A few years ago, we started to take an interest in the effect the food we eat has on how we feel, and it's safe to say that at the time we felt somewhat bewildered. New research promoted 5:2 and LCHF diets everywhere and were touted by overconfident health experts, which made it just about impossible to sift through all the advice and findings. One day we got fed up and launched a blog to try to make some sense of all the concepts—on our own.

Actually, things didn't begin quite like that. A few months earlier, we were in Helsingborg (a coastal city in the south of Sweden) to have lunch with Stig Bengmark, a professor of medicine. Three mouthfuls into a beet burger, Stig cracked open the door to what was for us a totally new world.

Bengmark was Professor of Surgery at the University of Lund's Medical Faculty, in southern Sweden, from 1970 to 1994; he was also Chairman and Director of the Department of Surgery at the Lund University Hospital from 1970 to 1992. Many years ago, he realized that about 80 percent of the body's immune system is located in the gut (gastrointestinal tract), whereupon he decided to devote the remainder of his career to finding out how to optimize one's intestinal flora. Today, Stig is Honorary Visiting Professor at University College, London University, where his task is to conduct research and teach about the best conditions for health.

On second thought, things didn't quite happen like that, either. A few years earlier, we had both become parents for the first time; with the concurrent births of Ninni and Ludde, we realized that we were not immortal. The sudden feeling of responsibility for someone else's life, along with wanting to always be there for them, resulted in months of nightly sessions Googling diseases, symptoms, and information on how to stay healthy, active, and strong forever. Somewhere amid all this anxiety, an interest was sparked on how much we ourselves can influence things by what we eat.

This book is a compendium of what we have learned. After blogging day and night for two years, it's time to summarize, in plain and simple language, all the research we have posted on the blog—and to push it even further. Even though we have long known that we have billions of bacteria in our bodies, it has taken scientists only until quite recently to grasp how critical a rich and thriving intestinal flora is to our health. Today, gastrointestinal research is one of the hottest fields in science, and we are constantly acquiring new knowledge and a deeper understanding of the connection between bacteria, intestinal flora, and well-being.

Today, we are aware that intestinal flora exerts a very strong influence on how we feel. We know that the flora consists not only of good bacteria but also bad, potentially disease-causing bacteria. We are conscious that good and bad bacteria can be strengthened or weakened depending on what we eat. We know that an excess of bad bacteria contributes to chronic inflammation; and we also know that chronic inflammation can make us ill.

Lina

Mia

In this book, we'd like to show you the fundamental connection between intestinal flora, inflammation, and your health. More important, we want to show how you can influence your intestinal flora and the way you feel in the long run through your own food choices.

This is the story of how we got interested in the link between health and food and how, to our surprise, we ended up among intestinal bacteria. Without Professor Stig, we would both still be at our old jobs (and still making a salary!). We'd also like to take the opportunity here to thank all the other science journalists, physicians, and scientists whom we've had the pleasure to get to know over the past few years. Thank you, everyone—without you, this book would have ended up being a simple haiku.

So, let's start from the beginning.

THE INTESTINAL FLORA'S COMMANDMENTS

Per the Food Pharmacy:

01. Focus on what you can eat, instead of what you must avoid eating.

02. Enjoy lots of different and colorful raw vegetables.

03. Eat meat sparingly.

04. Gorge on leafy greens.

05. Drink a green smoothie daily.

06. If you eat fish, opt for wild-caught varieties.

07. Eat slowly and chew thoroughly.

08. Skip processed foods.

09. Seek out organic food.

10. Increase foods' nutritional values by sprouting and fermenting them.

11. Lower the temperature by a few notches.

12. Choose your fats wisely.

Yummy

13. Add some zing to your food with herbs and spices.

14. Teach yourself and your kids to get comfortable without sugar.

15. Become a nutrient hunter (and avoid "fillers").

16. Give your body a chance to rest now and then with periodic fasting.

17. When you feel stressed out, take a deep breath and try to focus on the positives of life.

18. Move your body often!

19. Let food be your main source of nutrients, but feel free to give it a boost of added vitamin D, omega-3, and synbiotics.

20. Relax, and don't be too hard on yourself. That is the most important commandment of all.

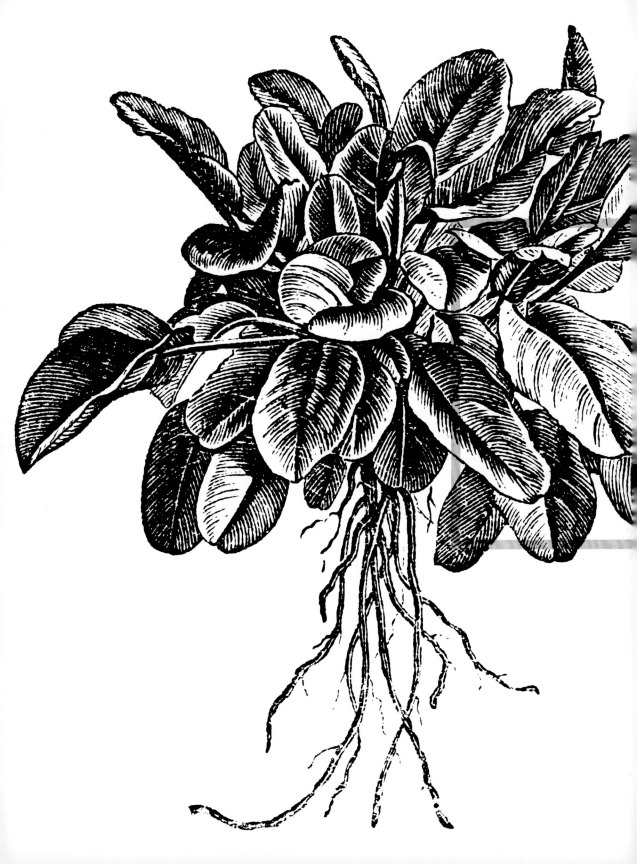

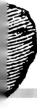

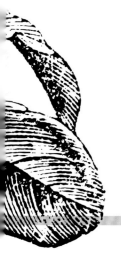

PLATO'S PLATE MODEL

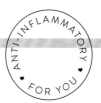

LET US TELL YOU ABOUT Plato before we delve deeper into intestinal bacteria and inflammation. (Well, not exactly "us"; it's Lina who will tell you about Plato. Mia is going to take this opportunity to paint her nails.)

Plato was born in Athens a few hundred years BC. He was a Greek philosopher, mathematician, and author, as well as the father of Platonism, which has contributed in many ways to Western philosophy. One example of Plato's legacy is his idealism, which is part of the foundation of mathematical philosophy. Well, you can see for yourself that Plato wasn't a few sandwiches short of a picnic.

A big part of Plato's philosophy is known as Plato's theory of ideas or forms. His theory encompasses two worlds, namely 1) the ideal (the perfect idea), and 2) the physical realm. According to Plato, nothing can exist in life without there also being a corresponding perfect idea (eternal, unchanging) of the same kind, in the world of ideas and forms.

For example:
When you walk past a vegetable garden and notice a potato, you think *potato* (if you don't, make an appointment to see an eye doctor). You still recognize, with 100 percent certainty, that this is just a potato, even if it's green and has begun sprouting. Plato says that this is because there is an ideal potato that all the potatoes in the real, tangible world strive to become, which is the reason you'd recognize the tuber as a potato, even if it were old and wrinkled.

– But Lina my dear, what does an old spud have to do with our book?

Mia screws the cap back onto the bottle of nail polish and blows on her nails. Lina looks at her.

– Hang on, I'm getting to the point soon.

Admittedly, Plato was mostly interested in mathematics, politics, and philosophy and not in potatoes, but we feel nonetheless that we can draw parallels with our relationship to food. Simply put, we could say that if the research and science presented in this book is in the realm of ideas, then we—our food-rejecting children and us and our cravings—are part of the real, material world. There exists an ideal, but there's also a reality, which we often surrender to.

For instance, let's say that all current research on food suggests that our intestinal flora would be at its happiest if we consumed twenty-two pounds of kale every day. We could call this "Plato's Plate Model," i.e., the idea of the perfect plate. In this ideal world, we would always eat twenty-two pounds of kale a day; however, in the real world that might end up being too big a challenge. First, most of us would probably find it difficult, not to mention a total drag, to choke down that much kale every day; and even if we were obstinate enough to try it, kale could be out of season, or the grocery store could be sold out. Second, we are humans and we have senses; if you add senses to the mix you'll end up with a real mess. You'll be attracted to the sight of a beautiful chocolate cake. Your sense of smell will be entranced by the aroma of freshly baked bread. The sound of a cork being pulled out of a bottle of wine will conjure up feelings of vacation and relaxation. Suddenly, there you are, gorging on a big piece of cake, working your way through a baguette, and downing several glasses of Bourgogne—even though none of these items are featured on Plato's Plate.

Mia looks up from her coral nails.

– Wow, I'd love a glass of wine . . .

– Yes, but that just proves my point! Plato's idealism is all about how it's impossible to be perfect in the real world. It's totally normal that we are unable to resist temptations; what would life be without them?

There is a prolonged silence. We hear the sound of a car passing in the street.

Mr. Plato

Before we started blogging about intestinal flora and inflammation, we were 1) thoroughly ruled by our senses, and 2) quasi-hypochondriacs. At the first smell of cardamom, we'd devour two buns with nary a thought; as soon as we heard the sparks of a fire being lit, we'd rush over to the grill, our sticks laden with marshmallows at the ready.

Then we'd head home, flip open our laptops, and read about how the rates of disease were rising all over the world; about how bad sugar was for our children; about how we got nowhere near enough fiber in our diets; and about how we'd all collapse suddenly and die if we so much as looked at a slice of bacon. It felt as though our lives were part of one big health lottery, where all we could do was close our eyes tightly, cross our fingers, and hope that we or anyone else we knew wouldn't get sick.

But then we started to read and educate ourselves. The more we learned, the less we felt the grip of anxiety. Do you know why? Because knowing that there is an ideal we could strive for relieved us of our paranoia.

Slowly but surely, we realized that we might not just be part of one big health lottery after all, and that there is a compass out there. With that in mind, we suddenly gave ourselves permission to grab a snack to calm our senses. (Though things did get a bit out of hand—"Ahem, that's the fifth day in a row you're eating a slice of cake for dinner. That's not exactly the best for your intestinal flora.")

This is our reasoning:
1 Somewhere out there is a perfect plate (in the ideal world).
2 We know that not every meal from here on out will compare favorably to the perfect plate (but that's okay, since we live in the real world).
3 But we will aim for the perfect plate, and we will try our best.

In other words, the research presented in this book is not a religion one must follow blindly. It is an ideal world we can keep in the back of our minds as we make our way through the real world full of cynical children, candy cravings, bellyaches, hunger pangs, broken hearts, and reward systems.

Another important thing to keep in mind is that what's in this book is not etched in stone. If we could have assembled every physician, scientist, and journalist we have interviewed and been inspired by in one big room, they would have seen eye-to-eye on many things but would have also disagreed on quite a few issues, too—that's a given. Research on intestinal flora is still in its infancy, but hopefully this book will give you a good picture of how food affects intestinal flora and show you in which direction the research is headed.

Learning about intestinal flora has been fun, but also a lot of work. Most of it is very logical, and it's great to realize that there are so many things we can do to affect our bodies. However, it's also a lot of work, because, well, it's frustrating to realize that a lot of the stuff many of us consume daily makes us unwell, both physically and mentally. We live in a world that has completely lost its footing, and in the race to make food cheaper to manufacture, the food industry has made us dependent on a diet that our bodies are ill equipped for, which includes processed foods lacking in fiber, antioxidants, and minerals and that are loaded with added sugars, pesticide residues, and unhealthy fats. Add to that the easy availability of a huge range of convenience food, and we have the first generation in human history that is literally eating itself to death.

Even so, we generally feel that our bodies are fantastic. With help from Plato's philosophy, we have come to realize that if we simply tune in to what our bodies require and make sure to give them plenty of nourishment each day, they will weather most storms. Select a few of the book's recipes and start making them at even intervals, and you'll be well on your way. Concentrate on all the wonderful things you'll be giving your body rather than what you are giving up, and your stress will disappear. In the real world, we don't agonize over eating an ice cream or that last margarita we drank. Sure, it won't strengthen our intestinal flora, but if there is something we have learned, it is that intestinal flora does not thrive on anxiety. We suggest, once and for all, that we lay to rest all of our health worries and guilty consciences!

– How about it Mia, is it time for a small, welcome drink yet?
Mia stands up and straightens her velour sweatpants.
– You bet!

FOOD PHARMACY'S WELCOME SHOT

(makes 1 glass)

²/₅ cup (100 ml) juice of your choice (if you're hard core, go for plain water)

1 tbsp ground turmeric

½ tsp ground black pepper

1 tsp ground cinnamon

1 pinch ground cloves

1 tbsp apple cider vinegar

1 tbsp olive oil

1 tbsp freshly squeezed lemon juice

We've drunk quite a few shots over the years, but—hand on heart—we've never had one that tastes like this. It was concocted by Professor Stig Bengmark, and he drinks one every day.

Mix and drink 1–2 times a day. Cheers!

Sometimes it can be difficult for the body to take in turmeric, so it's a good idea to drink it mixed with black pepper or chili or cayenne pepper, which helps absorb it.

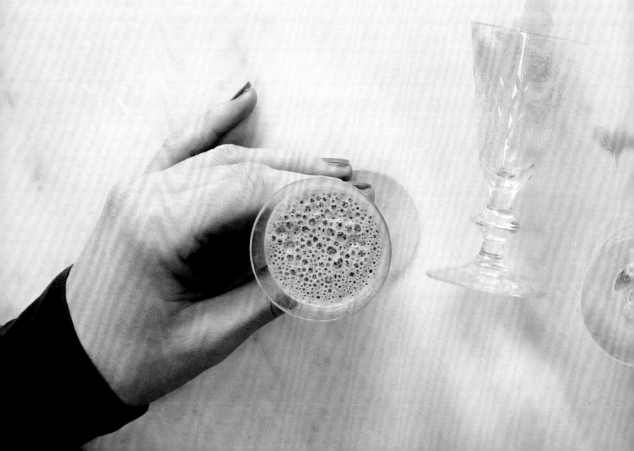

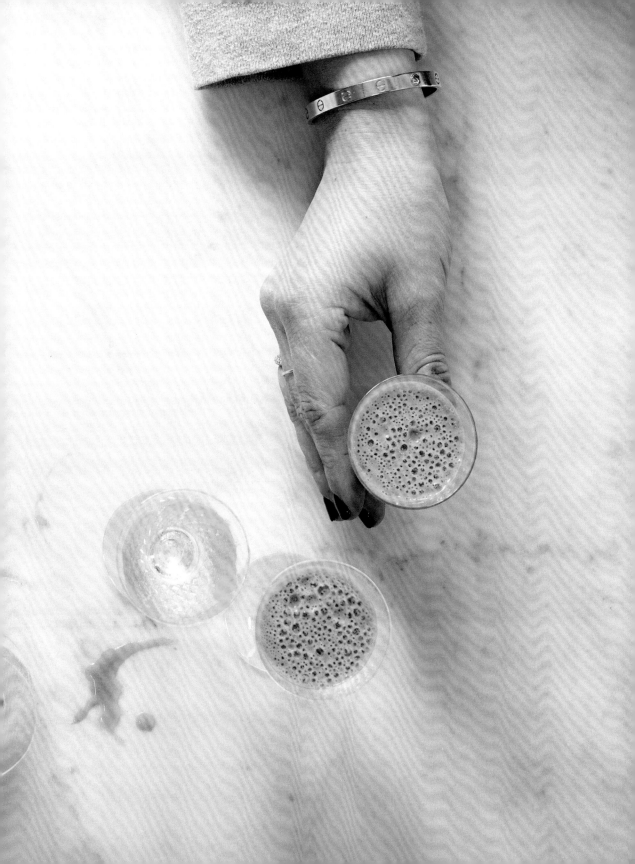

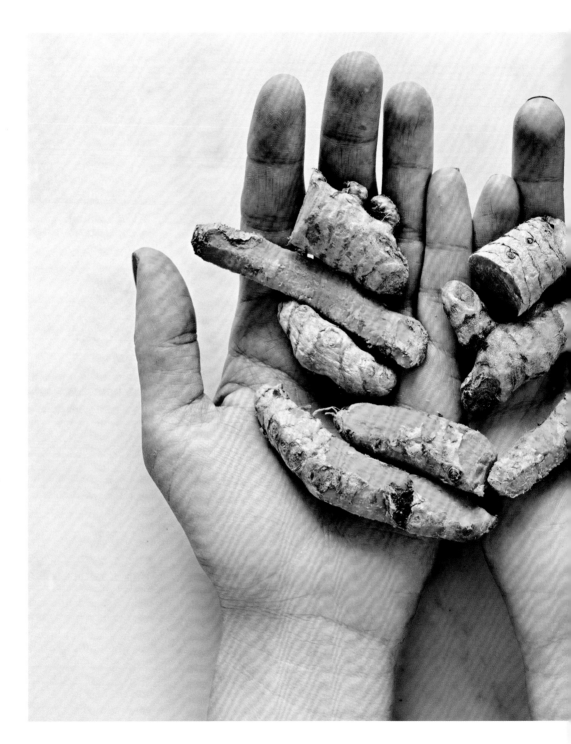

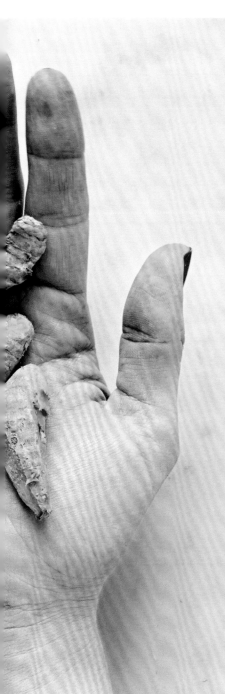

TURMERIC

One day, if we ever have the pleasure of meeting each other, you should know that it's perfectly okay to sneak a peek at our yellow hands. Considering their color, there are only two conclusions you might safely draw: either 1) we are heavy smokers, or 2) we love turmeric. (*The correct answer can be found at the bottom of this page.)

Turmeric is one of the most anti-inflammatory herbs in existence. One of the most inflammation-causing genes is COX-2, and scientists have worked for decades to discover a drug that can inhibit it. So far, all the drugs that have been pitted against COX-2 have had too many side effects. However, turmeric has shown itself to be a strong and nontoxic COX-2 inhibitor.

Professor Stig likes to think of turmeric as containing a small, complete soccer team of strong anti-inflammatory antioxidants called curcumenoids. He compares turmeric to the superstar Argentine soccer player Maradona. However, turmeric is also a team player and needs the other antioxidants to be present to play a winning game.

It can be difficult to find fresh turmeric. We love it both fresh and in powder form!

The correct answer is of course 2) we love turmeric.

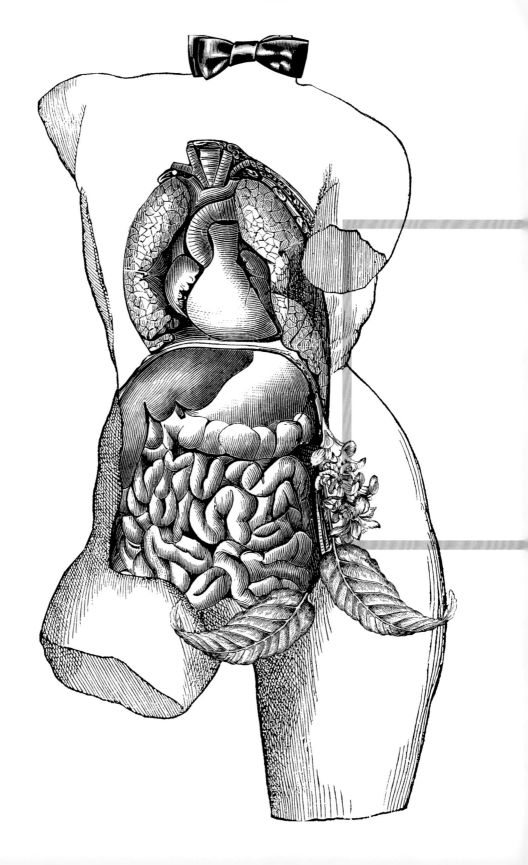

INFLAMMATION —THE UNWELCOME GUEST

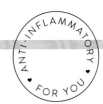

BY NOW, most of us have come to realize that the food we eat can have a direct effect on how we feel. Some have discovered how much more alert and energized we are by ingesting certain foods, while we get bellyaches from other foods. But honestly, can broccoli, kale, and raspberries help us fight off illness? Is it true that a sizeable daily dose of turmeric can keep us healthy? Isn't that taking things a bit far?

According to current research, it isn't. We live in very exciting times—every other day uncovers new studies related to intestinal flora and inflammation, their results demonstrating that by changing our lifestyle and what we eat, we can play an active role in preventing an array of maladies such as infections, cardiovascular disease, high blood pressure, achy joints, MS (Multiple Sclerosis), diabetes, headaches, ADHD (Attention Deficit Hyperactivity Disorder), skin problems, sleep disorders, and cancer. The fact is, the food we chomp down on makes a difference deep down at life's cellular level. In the same way that excess sugar and processed foods can make us sick, fiber-rich vegetables, colorful spices and grains, and cereals rich in antioxidants can help us stay healthy and vital.

Before getting to know our own in-house professor, Stig Bengmark, we used to call ourselves "positive hypochondriacs." We thought often about illnesses and called the health hotline a bit more often than the average person; yet we still looked to the future with optimism.

It's easy to make light of one's preoccupation with health—that nagging worry that sickness may strike out of the blue—but it's not so easy to live with. To be honest, not many afflictions have escaped our paranoia over the years, including cancer, cardiovascular disease, diabetes, rheumatism, and a few other choice ailments. Then we met Stig. That's when our obsession with inflammation began.

You're probably thinking: *Inflammation? That doesn't sound so bad.*

Nope, and it took us by surprise, too. We were worried about lumps and bumps and stiff joints, and then here comes Stig, throwing a big pile of scientific articles in front of us, insisting that inflammation is the real villain.

And he's not going on about inflamed cuticles, either; he's talking about *chronic inflammation.*

SO, WHAT IS CHRONIC INFLAMMATION?

First, we need to understand the difference between common and chronic inflammation.

The clinical definition of *inflammation* is "the body's attempt at self-protection; the aim being to remove harmful stimuli." Common inflammation isn't particularly complicated—it is simply the body's natural defense against foreign invaders such as bacteria, toxins, or a virus. The affected area attracts immune system cells—white blood cells—from the blood, and those cells emit different substances to root out the cause of the inflammation and repair any harm caused to the body's cells.

The body is a total pro at protecting itself against bacterial and viral invaders, and in those instances inflammation is a good thing. Except in one case: chronic inflammation. The word *chronic* means that it is long-lasting and persistent. Chronic inflammation is as damaging to the body as a run-of-the-mill, short-lived inflammation is beneficial. Chronic inflammation is silent and vicious; it differs from a common, acute case of inflammation in that it is as discreet as the Millenium Series' Lisbeth Salander, and it can be just as challenging to deal with. The signs are there, but they're so subtle that their little warning bells might be difficult to hear, at least at the onset.

SIGNS OF CHRONIC INFLAMMATION

Unexplained fatigue
Trouble sleeping
Headaches
Hair loss
Premature graying
Dandruff
Acne
Unexplained breakouts and red, blotchy skin
Dry eyes
Brittle nails
Dry mouth or excess saliva
Decreased libido
Irregular periods
Unexplained chronic constipation or diarrhea
Unexplained osteoporosis
Frequent, unexplained infections and influenza
Frequent mental depression
Unexplained shortness of breath
Sweaty feet and sweaty palms

Uh-oh, oh no!

Don't panic—exhibiting the above symptoms doesn't necessarily mean that you suffer from chronic inflammation. Sweaty palms might be from nervousness, and a sudden shortness of breath is a common reaction to falling head over heels in love.

But since we know that chronic illness is preceded by chronic inflammation, and that the rate of these chronic diseases is increasing, it is not unreasonable to conclude that many of us could be walking around with chronic inflammation and be completely unaware of it. It's enough to make one think long and hard about countries that have embraced the Western diet and that are also experiencing surging rates of allergies, rheumatism, ADHD, diabetes, and cancer.

However, if so many of us have chronic inflammation, why is it that we can't feel it? Maybe we think it's no big deal to feel constipated, or to have breakouts, or to suffer from unexplained fatigue. Perhaps we have simply learned to live with our aches and pains and believe it's the normal run of things. It would be a shame if that were the case, knowing as we do now that chronic inflammation is an important factor in chronic illness, and that today's research indicates that if one develops a chronic illness, the odds of suffering a second and third ailment are greater. However, what has not been understood yet is why the disease process begins with cancer in one individual, starts with diabetes in someone else, and triggers Alzheimer's disease in yet another.

HOW DOES CHRONIC INFLAMMATION EMERGE?

Let's go back to the body.

Alzheimer's disease, type 2 diabetes, and cancer are some of the most common chronic diseases.

Chronic inflammation develops when the immune system is exhausted. Each time we take a breath we inhale about 500 ml (1 pint) of oxygen into our lungs. From the lungs, the oxygen is sent out via the bloodstream to our blood cells, which need oxygen to produce energy. Not only is vital energy made during this process, something called *free radicals* is also produced, which in large quantities can damage the body's cells and cause inflammation.

The formation of free radicals also happens through our lifestyle choices. Let say, for instance, that you don't take care of yourself—you eat a bad diet, suffer from stress, don't exercise, and smoke. A great many free radicals would be formed in the cells, too many for your body to guard itself against. This wears out your immune system, and chronic inflammation ensues.

Antioxidants can effectively disarm those free radicals. As the name implies, antioxidants defend us from the damage inflicted by free radicals on the body's cells. A small number of antioxidants are produced by our bodies, but as we age our ability to make antioxidants decreases. From about twenty-five years of age, the body stops producing its own antioxidants entirely, which is why it's critical that we obtain them through our food in the form of vegetables, fruit, and berries. In the next chapter, we'll show you that there are two types of bacteria to be found in the gut—good and bad bacteria—but we can already reveal at this point that it's the good bacteria in our gut that extracts antioxidants from the food we eat. This is why we can easily help our body defend itself

Fig. #1

FACTORS THAT AFFECT YOUR HEALTH

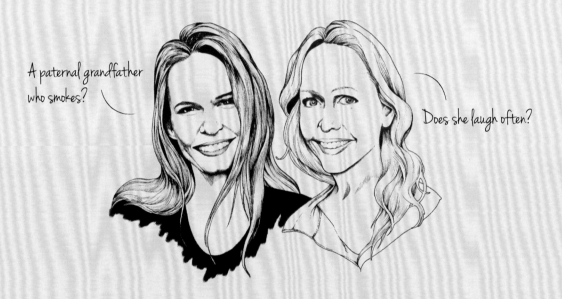

Does your father go to the gym?   What did your paternal grandmother eat when she was growing up?

Do we smoke?   Do we get enough sleep?   Is your maternal grandfather a couch potato?

A paternal grandfather who smokes?

Does she laugh often?

Do we always find an excuse to eat unhealthy meals?   Are our intimate relationships fulfilling?

Does your mother take a lot of antibiotics?   Do we consume enough antioxidants, fiber, vitamins, and minerals?

Did we eat a lot of processed foods and candy while growing up?   Are we under a lot of stress?

What was your maternal grandmother's lifestyle while she was pregnant with your mom?

against free radicals by gorging on large salads and delicious smoothies, thereby boosting our levels of good gut bacteria. More about this a little further along in the book.

GREAT NEWS! GENES HAVE FAR LESS INFLUENCE THAN WE ORIGINALLY THOUGHT.

In the US, the average life expectancy is 81.64 years for women and 76.73 years for men, but research has shown that, genetically speaking, humans have the capacity to grow much older than this. Some scientists even believe that the world's first two-hundred-year-old person has already been born. We have given this a lot of thought, but for us the most important thing has never been how old we'll get to be in years, but rather our quality of life. Because while life expectancy increases, we're also witnessing an increase in chronic diseases. If you can't enjoy them, what's so great about living all those extra years?

Human cells contain approximately 25,000 genes. According to Professor Stig, if your genes are a huge piano with 25,000 keys, then the sound of the inflammation symphony will depend on how you treat the keys. The more vitamins, antioxidants, minerals, and good fats you use to grease the keys, the more beautiful the melody. The more you mistreat the keys with bad food, lack of physical activity, medications, toxins, and stress, the faster Mozart will turn in his grave.

Research shows that there are thousands of factors contributing to chronic inflammation. Your genetic heritage is affected by everything—from how your paternal grandfather lived when he was a child to how your mother felt before and during her pregnancy. Was your paternal grandfather a smoker? Was your mother stressed out during her pregnancy? The answers to these questions can explain why you are who you are, why you feel like you do, and how long you will live—but only up to a point. The most significant impact is made by something entirely different: yourself.

Take a look at the picture on the left. Differences in life expectancy can largely be explained by inherited genes, but the good news is that we can influence those inherited traits via our

It's never too late, even if you've lived on junk food every day! A radical change of lifestyle and nutritional habits will soon yield the best chances for a healthy life.

lifestyle. The way we live is the most important factor in whether we will go on to develop chronic inflammation and chronic diseases or not. If you believe that your lifestyle exerts a greater influence on your health rather than your genes, and that your lifestyle can change some of your genetic heritage, then the two lovely ladies in the middle of the picture on page 24 have significant influence over the amount of inflammation in the body.

Fact
Current scientific research indicates that many diseases can be eliminated purely through diet.

Fact
As many as 30–35 percent of all cancers (depending on the type of cancer) are believed to be linked to what we eat.

Fact
Even someone who is otherwise very healthy can become sick, but they can probably improve their prognosis and lessen their risk of getting ill again by the way of a healthy lifestyle.

The ski lift stops with a sudden jolt. Mia removes one glove.
  – Things like that turn me on.
  Lina mulls it over.
  – Me too, but all the same, anyone can be unlucky and get sick.
  – Well, obviously! But I was thinking that might be a comfort, even for those who are not well, to know that in many cases, a change of lifestyle can improve the odds of getting better. No one was there to give my mother any dietary advice in all her years of her illness. I just feel so sad thinking about this now.
  Lina removes her ski goggles.
  – Do you remember that senior consultant in oncology who devotes all his free time to informing people about how diet can fight illness?
  – Totally!
  – When I interviewed him, he told me that it is not his contractual duty with the county council medical institution to inform his cancer patients about diet and nutrition, and that his time with his patients is so limited and booked up that he only has time to inform them about medical treatment.
  – Oh wow, that's horrible . . .

Juni, Mia's daughter, interrupts.
– Mom, why is the lift not moving?
Mia looks worriedly behind her.
– I don't know, honey . . .
The sun is setting lower behind the spruce tops. Mia realizes she needs to pee.

And with that we're ready to jump to the next chapter. The time has come to move down the body—because chronic inflammation starts further down, in the colon. Go to the kitchen and fix yourself our wonderful anti-inflammatory super smoothie, which you'll find on the next page, and then we'll continue as soon as you're back. In the ideal world, we drink a whole quart of this stuff every day, while in the real world it might just be a tad less.

PROFESSOR STIG'S ANTI-INFLAMMATORY SMOOTHIE

(Makes 1 pitcher)

10½ oz (300 g) kale

1 quart (1 liter) water

2 avocados

⁴/₅ cup (200 ml) rolled oats

1 half lemon, peeled

¾-inch (2 cm) nub fresh ginger, peeled

We enjoy this smoothie almost every day. It's full of antioxidants that fight free radicals. And it contains beneficial fibers. And good fats. And lots of hot ginger.

Mix. Pour into a glass. Drink up.

If the smoothie is too "green" for your taste, try adding in an apple.

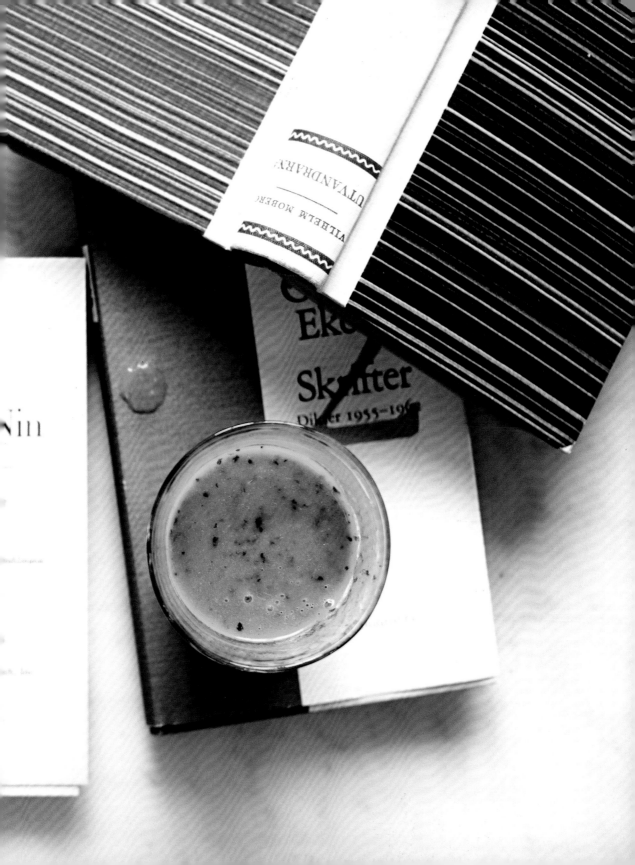

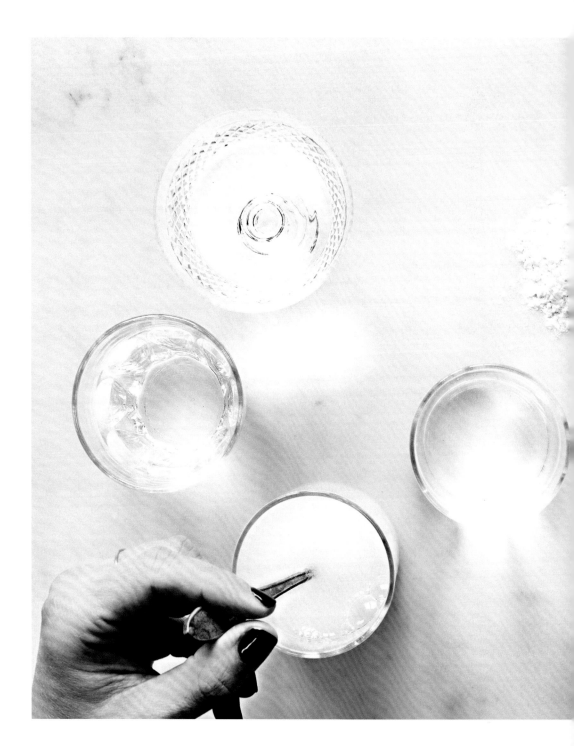

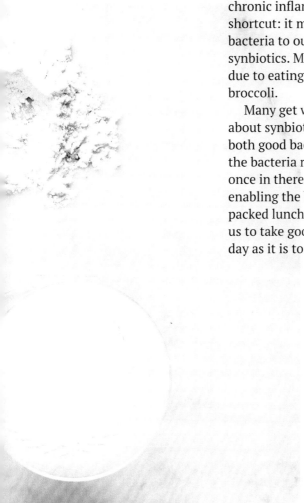

Food Pharmacy's Favorite #2

SYNBIOTICS

Just as we're beginning to understand gut flora and chronic inflammation, Professor Stig lets us in on a shortcut: it might be a good idea to add some good bacteria to our diet in the form of probiotics or synbiotics. Most of us today have poor intestinal flora due to eating too many potato chips and not enough broccoli.

Many get what probiotics are all about, but what about synbiotics? They are supplements that have both good bacteria (probiotics) and fiber. Fiber helps the bacteria reach all the way down into the colon, and once in there the fiber becomes food for the bacteria, enabling the bacteria to grow and multiply. It's like a packed lunch for the probiotics. It is now as natural for us to take good bacteria and fiber in supplements each day as it is to change into clean underwear.

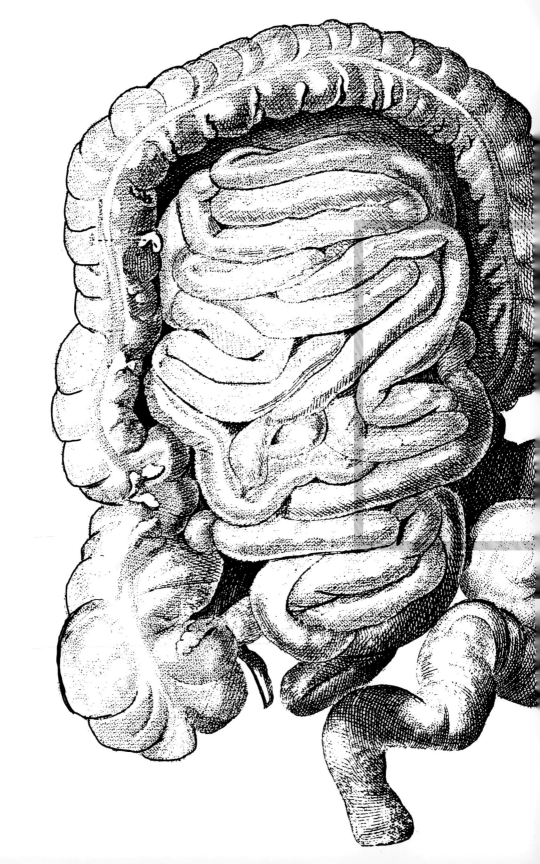

3

THE BATTLE OF THE GASTROINTESTINAL TRACT

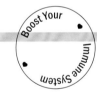

Boost Your Immune System

WHAT HAPPENED? We had never heard the words "intestinal flora" uttered before we started blogging, and now we say it almost every day. What's up with that?

Lina: *Would you like some broccoli in your smoothie?*
The kids: *Yeah! That will make our intestinal flora happy!*

Mia: *What, are we* only *having sauerkraut for dinner? Don't we have something to go with it?*
Lina: *Only sauerkraut. The intestinal flora is an entire ecosystem that needs to be fed daily.*

Emil, Mia's son: *Do we really have the energy to make dinner tonight? Why don't we just order pizza?*
Mia: *No thanks, my little man. I need to think of our intestinal flora.*

SOME GOOD NEWS AND SOME BAD NEWS

Professor Stig was a very successful surgeon and one of the innovators and pioneers in hepato-pancreato-biliary abdominal surgery before he started his research on intestinal flora. We're not talking about small and trivial procedures here; oftentimes the entire pancreas or big sections of the liver had to be removed. Unfortunately, it didn't always turn out as well as Stig would have hoped. Or, more accurately, the surgery would go well, but afterward the patients were often hit with difficult infections, which troubled Stig enormously.

During the 1950s, he suddenly saw things from a different angle. He had asked a young surgeon to study the last eighty-one big liver surgeries. One day, without warning, the young physician knocked on the door and told Stig that he had some good and some bad news. Stig ushered him into the room and told him to start with the bad news. A little awkwardly, the young doctor told him that in a third of the patients for whom antibiotics should have been prescribed for the week after the surgery, as per the praxis of the day, the medication had not been given.

Stig was furious and fuming. How was this even possible at one of Sweden's top-notch university hospitals? Then, the young doctor smiled broadly.

But Stig, he said, I have some good news, too! All the infections we found were in the patients who had received their antibiotics. There were no infections among the patients who had not been given the medication.

There and then, a new thought sprang to Stig's mind: what if the antibiotics had knocked out the patients' immune system? A few years later, the Norwegian physician and professor of immunology, Per Brandtzaeg, published a study that confirmed approximately 80 percent of the immune system is in the gastrointestinal tract, which was enormously encouraging to Stig. It gave him the necessary push to start searching for methods to restore intestinal flora after it has been destroyed.

And, well, so the story goes.

INTESTINAL FLORA IS VITAL

Without getting ahead of ourselves, we can start by noting that the key to staying healthy and free of inflammation and chronic illness is a well-functioning intestinal flora. Simply put, this flora is the bacteria and microorganisms that exist naturally in the intestine. In an adult, this is between 3.3 to 4.4 lb of bacteria. The intestine is a huge ecosystem containing several hundred different types of good and bad bacteria, which is an amount at least ten times greater than the number of body cells we have—approximately a hundred trillion. So, in that respect, you're actually more bacteria than human. Most of your immune defense (or immune system, as it is also called) is in the gut (gastrointestinal tract), a truly fascinating system that's built on a close collaboration between immune cells in the intestinal wall and your army of good intestinal bacteria. To fight inflammation, it is vital that only the good bacteria hook onto those immune cell receptors in the intestine. If the bad bacteria latch on to the receptors instead, you will have inflammation and lesser resistance against infection.

Even though the atmosphere in the gut is so influential to how we feel, it is still one of the most unchartered areas of our body. You might think it's a bit odd when you realize that 70 to 80 percent of our immune system is situated there. But in recent years, interest in gut and intestinal flora has positively skyrocketed. Scientific research shows that bacteria in the colon not only affects a long list of illnesses and other conditions, such as diabetes, allergies, asthma, MS (multiple sclerosis), autism, cardiovascular disease, and some cancers, but also that they communicate with the brain and can drive our body weight, personality, and even our behavior. There are far more links between our gut and our brain than we first knew, with some scientists going so far as to call the gastrointestinal tract "our second brain."

For example, it isn't simply too little exercise and too much food that makes us fat: research shows that obesity can just as often be caused by inefficient gut flora and inflammation. Some studies even suggest that intestinal bacteria can influence our feelings of hunger and push us to crave certain foods that make their specific strain stronger than other bacterial strains in the gut. Studies have been set up where slim subjects were given intestinal flora from overweight donors, the outcome being that the slim subjects became overweight. This demonstrates that bacteria can sway us and make us fat by tricking the brain into believing that we're hungry.

Another thing we found very interesting is the connection between intestinal flora and depression. Your risk of being diagnosed with clinical depression increases substantially if you suffer from chronic inflammation. By now it hasn't escaped anyone's notice that exhibiting a low level of the neurotransmitter *serotonin* is linked to depression and dejection. These days, the amount of prescriptions written for serotonin-boosting antidepressants (SSRI, Selective Serotonin Reuptake Inhibitors) is astronomical. Approximately more than one in ten Americans take antidepressants, and the rate at which those prescriptions are issued is rising faster still for young people and teenagers. Naturally, we were surprised to learn that only 5 to 10 percent of serotonin is found in the brain. Where is the remaining 95 percent hiding out? Answer: in the gastrointestinal tract. By the way, serotonin is not the only hormone made in the gut; intestinal flora is in fact a key player in the production of all the body's hormones, providing our organs with these very important substances.

We could go on about this, but we do have to end it somewhere. All these findings are overwhelming; it's even more head-spinning to realize that it wasn't that long ago when medical students and budding dieticians were taught that bacteria in the body didn't play an important function. Today, vigorous research is being conducted in that field, and new studies are continually proving how critical our intestinal flora is to both our physical and mental well-being.

Lina stops chopping.

– So, I read somewhere that an internationally known scientist is thinking of writing a thriller about someone attempting to seize power over the Earth by manipulating humans' intestinal flora. Imagine how much power these little buggers have over our bodies.

Mia gets up from her chair and walks over to the pot to taste the soup.

– Yes, and I saw on the news that one of Sweden's most respected nutrition experts said he couldn't believe his eyes when he began reading about the connection between intestinal flora and health—that almost all illnesses and health problems can be linked directly to the flora in our gut.

Mia takes another sip of the soup. Lina screws up her face and shudders.

– Did you just double-dip?

– Come again?

– That spoon? Did you just lick it before you put it back in the soup?

– No . . . well yes . . . maybe . . . ?

Lina snorts and starts chopping again.

THERE IS AN ALL-OUT WAR IN YOUR GASTROINTESTINAL TRACT

Almost one hundred years ago, the Danish scientist Christian Gram discovered that some bacteria absorbed color through their cell walls while others didn't. Since then, bacteria that soak up color have been called Gram-positive (Gram+), while the nonabsorbent bacteria are called Gram-negative (Gram-). Plainly put, Gram+ are bacteria that protect against illness, while Gram- are the nasty ones, bacteria that, among other things, produce the strongly inflammatory and disease-inducing *endotoxin* poison. Since almost all Gram+ bacteria are benign and most of the Gram- are detrimental to our health, we thought we would keep things simple by referring to Gram+ and Gram- as good and *bad* bacteria.

When we are at our peak, we have about a hundred billion (and a thousand different strains of) good bacteria in our gut that work full-time to extract beneficial substances for us. Ideally, there should be about one nasty bacteria per one million (1,000,000) beneficial ones, but with today's nutritional habits we are nowhere near this ratio. We are correct in asserting that there is war in our gastrointestinal tract—a conflict between our good Luke Skywalkers and evil Darth Vaders.

You can trust your good Luke Skywalkers—they're always ready to defend your health, so long as you give them the right fuel. When you eat raw vegetables, they start multiplying rapidly and form an army so big and powerful that it can swiftly beat back your Darth Vaders and inhibit the inflammation reaction in your body.

Problem is, the diet most of us subsist on today is more likely to strengthen our Darth Vaders than our Luke Skywalkers, and our good bacteria die out when there isn't enough food for them. If we chow down on potato chips and French fries all the time, we're fueling the Darth Vaders, who mow down everything in their path,

When we are at our peak, we have about a hundred billion (and a thousand different kinds of) good bacteria in our gut that work full-time at extracting beneficial substances for us. The goal is to pit one Darth against each Luke, but thanks to today's diet things aren't looking so good.

Lukes included, and as a result our intestinal flora is knocked out of balance, our immune system is weakened, and inflammation arises.

Let's look at things from a more positive viewpoint. The advantage of good bacteria is that when they exist in an environment in which they thrive, they're able to defend us from inflammation and disease-causing bacteria. We just need to give them enough nourishing food (vegetable fibers, antioxidants, minerals, and good fats), and they'll quickly grow strong and multiply.

Beneficial bacteria have many important tasks besides chasing out nasty bacteria. For example, they line the intestinal wall and ensure that toxins and other waste don't leak out into the bloodstream and into the rest of the body. Imagine that your gastrointestinal tract is like a long, winding, amusement-park water slide through your body, and that Luke's army extracts all the antioxidants, vitamins, amino acids, and minerals that you send down the chute to release nutrients into your body. Thanks to the slide's enclosed system, substances that Luke's army doesn't need or want—the debris, toxins, and dead bacteria—can simply leave the body.

By the way, is it only the two of us who have suddenly gotten the urge to give our Lukes a treat? We'll put some kale in the oven and keep on reading while it turns into chips.

Well-functioning intestinal flora decreases inflammation in the body, stimulates the body's own immune system, and protects against repeat infections, chronic illnesses, and premature aging.

LUKE SKYWALKER'S KALE CHIPS

(makes one baking sheet full)

In the ideal world, we make our own sesame milk and homemade nut butter all the time, but we can't quite get it together on a typical day when the kids are skateboarding through the living room. That's when we use grocery store shortcuts. However, you will never find kale chips among those quick-fixes. We happily make these from scratch at least once a week. They are very easy to make and scrumptious.

½ lb (250 g) kale

2 tbsp olive oil

Few pinches sea salt

Heat the oven to no higher than 175°F (80°C). Rinse the kale thoroughly and dry the leaves with a kitchen towel. Tear the kale into pieces the size of, let's say, a LEGO® figurine, and toss them for 1 to 2 minutes in a bowl with olive oil and sea salt. Spread the kale onto a baking sheet and leave it in the oven for about 40 minutes. The best is to leave the oven door slightly open. Remove the chips from the oven when they are crisp.

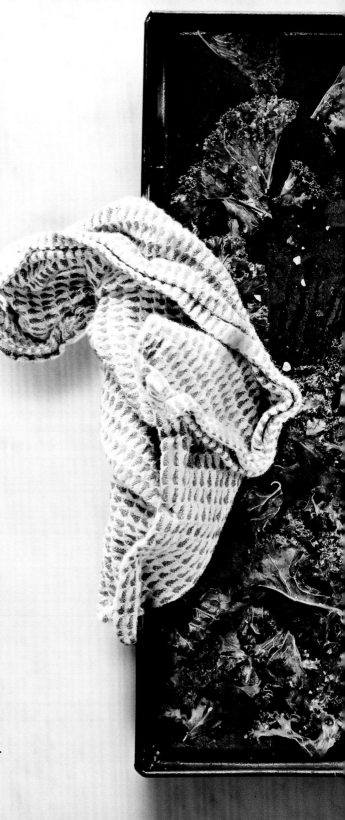

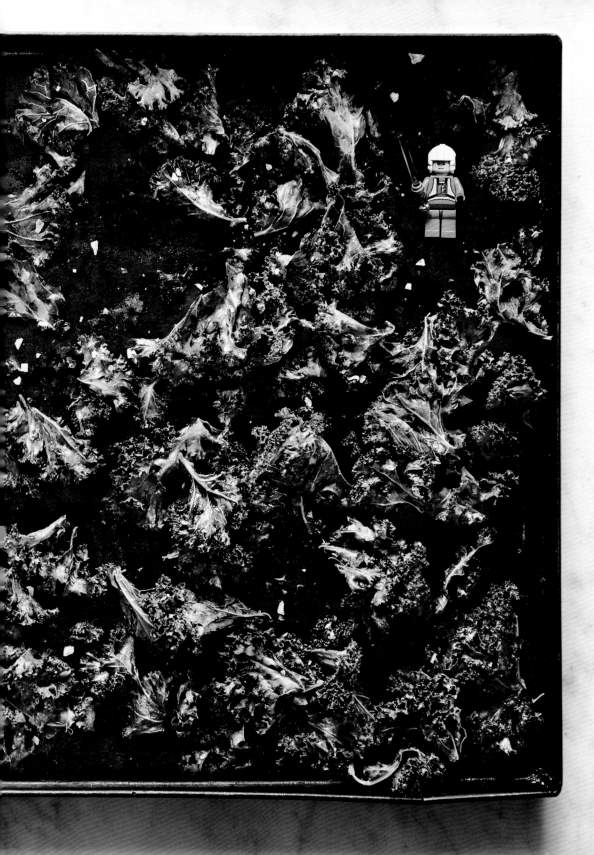

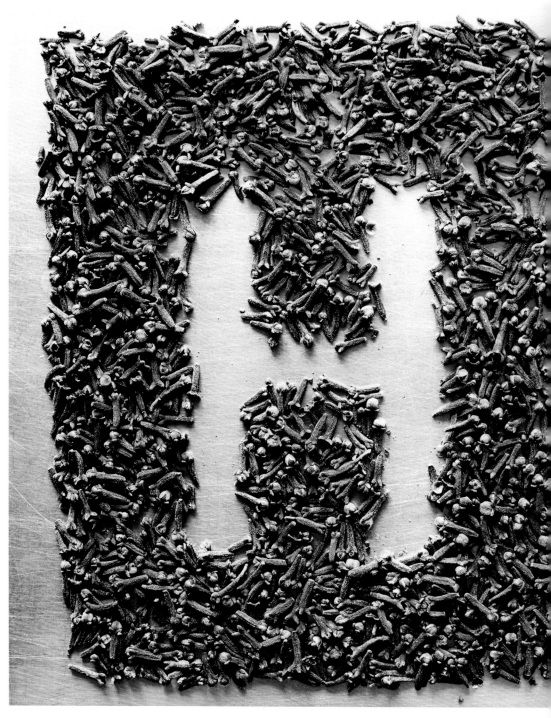

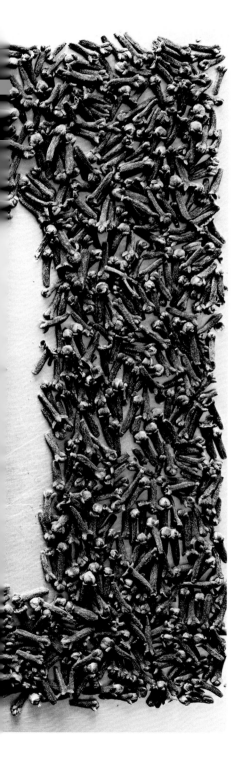

CLOVES

Cloves might make you think of snowmen, Christmas trees, and Bing Crosby, but for us they're the world's strongest antioxidant. Cloves are an Indonesian spice that has been part of Asian medicine for thousands of years, and they deserve to be used more often than just plugged into oranges to make pomander balls one measly month of the year. Instead, crush cloves with a mortar and pestle and then add them to your smoothie, soup, chutney, coffee, or tea.

Cloves have a rather pungent taste—our best tip is to mix them with other anti-inflammatory spices, such as cinnamon and ginger.

Cloves are world-famous for their strong anti-inflammatory, antiseptic, anesthetic (numbing), rubefacient (warming and soothing), and antiflatulent properties.

That last benefit is just a nicer way of saying that the spice works to prevent farting.

WHERE IN THE BODY IS FOOD ABSORBED?

Nutrients we ingest from food eventually leave the intestinal tract and make their way into the bloodstream to be moved to the body cells. However, the question is where are they absorbed—directly from the small intestine, or a few hours later from the large intestine (colon)?

Raw vegetables are exceptionally hard to digest, and as a result they travel all the way down to the colon. Once there, they dole out nutrients to our good Luke Skywalkers and defend us from inflammation. Unfortunately, most of the food we eat today is neither raw nor slow to digest. On the contrary, most of our daily food—white bread, pasta, and rice, for instance—is already taken up in the small intestine. Food that is processed, treated with pesticides, and lacking in fiber = a real cocktail of inflammation factors.

When we consume food that gets absorbed in the small intestine, our protective bacteria in the colon don't get any of the fiber-, mineral-, and antioxidant-rich nutrients they need. You'll recall that antioxidants are our body's foremost protectors against free radicals and that they guard us from inflammation, illness, and premature aging. Without those antioxidants, free radicals are free to wreak havoc. In short order, this means a lowered immune system that's plagued by lingering colds, and in the long run it could lead to worse. Food that is absorbed in the small intestine elevates blood sugar levels too fast, and this in turn overburdens our digestive organs—the liver and the pancreas—because they are put under stress when dealing with the excess sugar in the blood (which causes inflammation) as quickly as possible.

The stronger the color, the more abundant the antioxidants. That's why kale contains four to five times more antioxidants than white cabbage.

THE ENEMIES OF GASTROINTESTINAL FLORA

From the picture on the page to the right, we can see clearly how, in the Western part of the world, we have decimated large sections of our intestinal flora. Westerners (the yellow line) have lost 40 percent of their intestinal flora compared to the Yanomami, an indigenous population of the Amazon (the green line), and 20 percent compared to countries where the population consumes a diet somewhere between ours and the Yanomami's.

Fig. #2

AMOUNTS OF BACTERIAL STRAINS IN MICROBIOTA—DIFFERENT GEOGRAPHICAL AREAS

(Source: Clemente JC et al Science Advances 2015;1 (3)

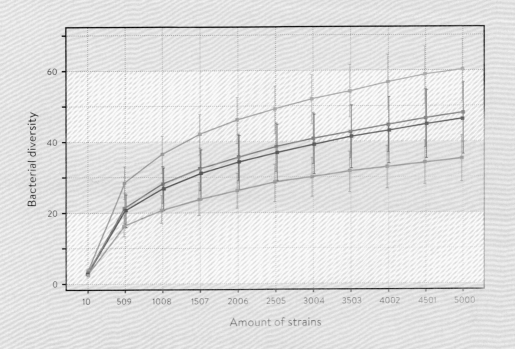

The Yanomami have lived without any contact with the modern world and have thus held on to their rich intestinal flora, which means that they hardly ever suffer from inflammatory conditions. In countries that have adopted a Western lifestyle, we can see high rates of chronic illness, which is caused by inflammation and bad intestinal flora. Processed food, along with little exercise and lots of stress, has depleted our intestinal flora and disturbed the balance of good and bad bacteria. Other studies show that today's children and young people often have difficulty building protective intestinal flora because, among other things, they don't eat a diet that encourages its growth. Projections indicate that rates of most chronic diseases will triple or even quadruple by the year 2050. In Sweden, research has shown that every other Swede will be affected by cancer at some point during his or her lifetime (currently, the ratio is one out of three).

A little while back we briefly mentioned another major threat: antibiotics. Aside from knocking out the good bacteria in the intestinal flora, excessive use of antibiotics has led to emerging problems with multidrug-resistant bacteria. This is called antibiotic resistance, and it is one of the biggest dangers facing our health today. Antibiotic resistance means that bacteria have developed to a point where no antibiotic can fight it. As modern-age travelers crisscross the planet, antibiotic resistance is becoming a global concern. For instance, antibiotic-resistant bacteria that develops in India could quickly affect someone in America, and ominous forecasts show that more people will die from multidrug-resistant bacteria than from cancer within the next twenty years. Scientists warn us that if we don't turn this situation around, multidrug-resistance will be the main cause of mortality by 2050.

So, use caution with antibiotics. If you're in a situation in which you need to take a course of antibiotic drugs, boost your Lukes with supplements of good bacteria (i.e., probiotics or synbiotics) over the course of treatment, as well as for a few days after you finish your medication. Feel free to add an extra spoonful of fermented vegetables to each meal, and eat more raw vegetables than you typically would.

EPIGENETICS—A SCIENTIFIC REVOLUTION

Epigenetics is a topic that keeps today's researcher from every field of science busy, from cancer and cardiovascular disease to

It is commonly believed that a simple course of antibiotics can destroy up to 90 percent of beneficial intestinal flora.

diabetes and depression. Epigenetics is the link between DNA and the environment. We have already touched on this in the past chapter, but it bears repeating: You have inherited a set of genes from your parents that you will always have to grapple with, but through your choice of lifestyle you may have a say in how they come into play. What is so interesting is that scientists have only recently started to understand that your intestinal flora could be one of the determining factors of whether a gene is activated or not.

By studying why twins who were raised apart during childhood could develop completely different illnesses—even though their genetic makeup is identical—it was discovered that the environment triggered the gene in one twin but not the other. Perhaps you're underwhelmed by this finding, but within the scientific community, it was akin to a *revolution* that challenged Darwin's theory of evolution, as well as old school facts about heredity and environment.

Food enters the picture here, too. Studies show that antioxidants can determine if a gene responsible for a certain illness is activated or not, simply by protecting that gene from an attack by free radicals. Stress, drugs, exhaust fumes, and exercise are all factors that can influence gastrointestinal flora, but eating right is one of the simplest, quickest, and most effective ways to improve your gut flora and counteract inflammation. If you switch from living on take-out, frozen pizza, and beer to eating a diet with a wide variety of vegetables, you can quickly move from the "at-risk" column for chronic illness to suddenly showing no warning signs of impending illness at all. You can improve your chances as soon as today! Epigenetics is constantly in flux. If you know that you have inherited a dicey genetic profile, you can affect the outcome with lifestyle modifications. You are not powerless, even if you have inherited a few not-so-stellar genes. Many scientists believe that in the future we will even be able treat chronic conditions, and tailor our lifestyle to our genes, to help prevent genetic diseases.

So that's it. You now have three choices:
1 Burn this book and commence bingeing on marshmallows.
2 Feel completely depressed due to your bad diet, but keep on reading.
3 Sneak a peek at the kale chips in the oven (remove them if they are just about ready) and accept the challenges in the next chapter.

What would Luke have done?

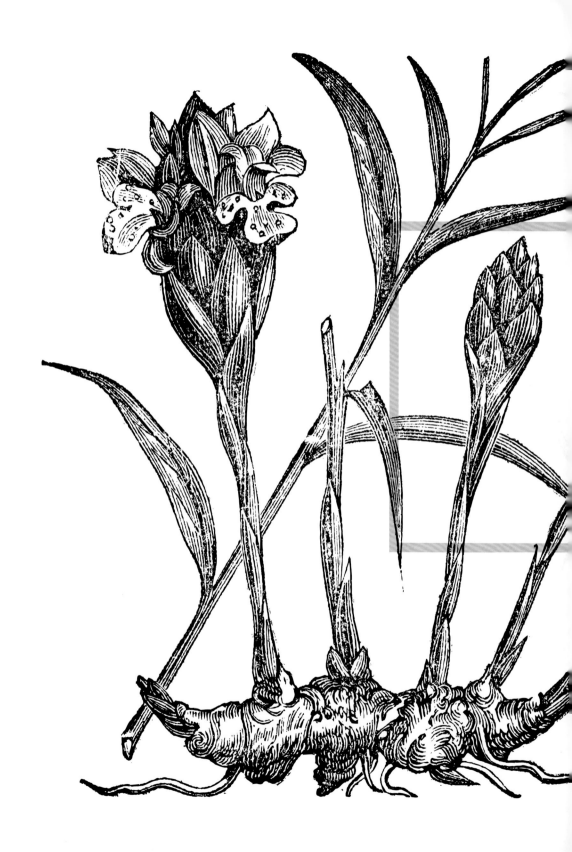

4

WELCOME TO THE ANTI-INFLAMMATORY KITCHEN

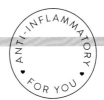

WELCOME TO THE ANTI-INFLAMMATORY KITCHEN. This is where we concentrate on enjoyment, from the first bite to the last. In our past lives, we believed there was a discrepancy between "good" and "good for you." How wrong we were.

We use good-quality, clean, raw ingredients that boost our Lukes: dark leafy greens, fatty fish, walnuts, buckwheat, avocado, and green bananas. We gorge on vegetables full of fiber, antioxidants, vitamins, and minerals, and devote a large section of our plate to foods in all colors of the rainbow. We enjoy a green smoothie every day, and let our body rest by practicing periodic fasting. We drink gallons of green tea. We prepare our food with love, and season it with oregano, turmeric, garlic, cloves, cinnamon, cardamom, and cocoa. We eat together with people who make us feel good, and finish the meal with high-quality coffee, dark chocolate, raspberries, red wine, and a good night's sleep.

What's that I hear? Was that your intestinal flora giving a big cheer? They really need to pipe down, because we're trying to talk here.

Now it's time for our six prescriptions. Each new chapter begins with a prescription: a summary of which foods make our intestinal flora happy and suppress inflammation. In the ideal world, we use all of them; in the real world, we all make our way from different starting points. It's important that you follow your own rhythm. Only you know what works best for you. Do everything at once, or concentrate on one chapter at a time. Or one recipe. Or just one word.

Cinnamon isn't just a spice that imparts a treat like sweetness to food; it also helps lower blood sugar. The cherry on top is that it's full of antioxidants and awesome for intestinal flora!

Common side effects from our prescriptions (reported in more than nine out of ten readers):
Happy gastrointestinal bacteria, halted inflammation, new ideas about diet, healthy gut flora, stable blood sugar, and lots of wonderful energy.

ATTENTION

Lisa falls apart at the table.

– Honestly, I just panic when I read your blog. I eat all the wrong things, and I feel faint just opening the web page. My husband has told me to stop reading Food Pharmacy.

Lina takes a mouthful of wine and puts her hand on Lisa's shoulder.

– How awful. The blog isn't meant to make you feel depressed. Why are you so anxious? All things considered, do you truly wish to change your eating habits?

– Well there's want, and then there's want . . . I feel like I should, but I haven't quite got the strength to do it. I just wish I could turn my cravings for cheese curds into cravings for green smoothies.

Mia laughs a little.

– If it's any comfort to you, I can tell you that I know exactly how you feel.

– Well, maybe so, but in my case it feels harder, because these aren't simple little tweaks that I need to make. Really, I need to change everything I eat. And I love my current diet. The only reason I would change anything is because you insist that what I eat isn't healthy for me.

Lina clears her throat.

– But Lisa, you don't have to change everything at once. Take it one step at a time. Start with just one small change. One healthy choice leads to another healthy choice, which then leads to . . .

Mia adds her bit.

– . . . a third, and soon enough you'll be a true health guru!

Lisa shuts her eyes. Mia fights a peppercorn that is stuck between her teeth.

– But come on, help me here—where do I begin?

– Have you read the book?

– Weeelll . . .

– Read the book again, and choose the changes you feel would be easiest for you to tackle. Maybe it's as simple as adding a green smoothie per day? That's how I started. It was much easier for me to add something than to take something away.

Lina interrupts.

– Hang in there, Lisa; don't give up. You know me: I've been exactly *where you are today. But if I can do it, you can do it.*

Lina gets up and heads toward the kitchen.

– Do you have bananas, raspberries, and coconut milk on hand?

– Yes . . .

– Give me three minutes and I will whip up the yummiest dessert for you. You can enjoy it every day when you crave something sweet. You can settle in on a Friday with this one. You can eat it for breakfast. You can bathe in it.

Lina goes into the kitchen and puts a banana, frozen raspberries, and coconut milk in a blender. She presses the start button, while Lisa picks up bits of Lisa, scattered over the dining-room table.

Sometimes it's so difficult to know where to begin that we don't start anything at all. There will be times when you realize you're not on a plan and might even have overdone things a little too much. Who cares? Concentrate on what you can do instead, and ignore what doesn't work for you. To be successful in the long run, you must focus on starting out from *your* situation, taking into account the unique possibilities and challenges you face. For instance, you can choose to concentrate on only one chapter of this book, and totally disregard the others. Or, you could follow all of it in one go, but only twice a week. Usually, one small change is better than several bigger ones that could trip you up because the obstacles are too great. Keep in mind that your real world needs to be an integral part of your journey.

TEACH YOURSELF AND YOUR CHILDREN TO GET COMFORTABLE WITHOUT SUGAR

(but enjoy treats every day)

In this chapter, you'll prepare a wonderfully delicious granola chock-full of anti-inflammatory cinnamon and cardamom, coconut flakes, and chopped almond and walnut. Why this recipe is so great: 1) It's super tasty, and 2) it doesn't contain any insulin-raising sugar (which is a change from so many other granolas). Just as coconut, nuts, and spices are treats for the good bacteria in the colon, sugar is fuel for the nasty bacteria. Sugar feeds Darth Vader's army and creates inflammation in the body. But you don't have to worry about that, so long as you follow this recipe.

LUKE SKYWALKER'S GRANOLA

(sorry, it only makes one baking sheet full)

⁴/₅ cup (200 ml) buckwheat groats

²/₅ cup (100 ml) pumpkin seeds

¹/₅ cup (50 ml) crushed flaxseeds

¹/₅ cup (50 ml) white sesame seeds

¹/₅ cup (50 ml) grated coconut flakes

²/₅ cup (100 ml) sweet almonds, chopped

²/₅ cup (100 ml) walnuts, chopped

2 tsp ground cinnamon

2 tsp ground cardamom

3 tbsp coconut oil, softened

We always lower the oven's temperature when we make granola. It takes a bit of time to cook, but it's infinitely kinder on the raw ingredients and intestinal flora.

Soak the buckwheat groats for 30 minutes. Heat the oven to 160°F (70°C). Mix the ingredients and spread them over a baking sheet lined with parchment paper. Let it bake for a few hours in the oven, stirring the contents from time to time. Remove the baking sheet from the oven when the granola feels dry and the whole kitchen smells of cinnamon.

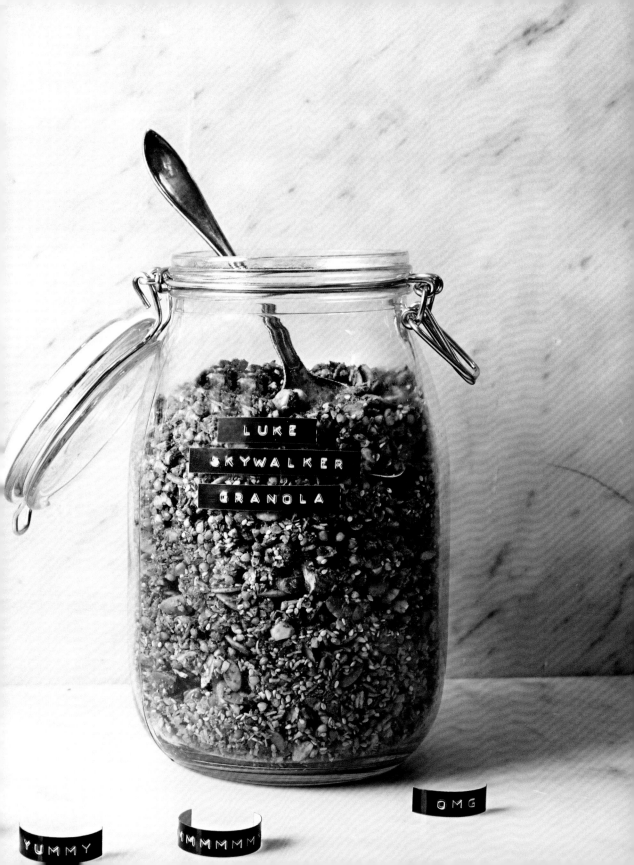

OUR SUGAR CV (CURRICULUM VITAE)

When we first got to know each other, gooey fudge cake was an integral part of our lives. We're talking literally here—it always had a spot between us. Most often, we'd sit on the floor in Mia's room, listening to Whitney Houston and enjoying our day's work straight from the baking pan. Sometimes we didn't even have a baking tin; we ate the batter straight from the mixing bowl. At times, we didn't even make a batter; we just poured sugar, butter, and cocoa directly into our mouths and gargled. That worked, too.

We could land a job in any candy store with our impressive sugar CV. Among other feats, we've gorged on two quarts of ice cream without getting sick, mixed cheap red wine with Coca-Cola, and now and again we've skipped dinner to dig into two-pound bag of pick 'n' mix candy. When I think of how much time we've spent thinking about salty licorice and cardamom rolls over the years, it's a minor miracle we ever learned anything in school.

You're not supposed to blame others for stuff, but hell yeah—we'll blame our parents. Sugar was considered a *good* thing when our moms and dads were growing up. It was lauded by nutritionists and marketed as the era's cheapest nutrient well into the 1950s. (Today, the average American consumes almost 150 pounds of sugar per year.)

By the way, this is probably the era when Lina's maternal grandma started to sprinkle sugar onto eggs, and Mia's maternal grandma served cookies for breakfast. Of course, you had to be a bit careful with sugar because it could give you cavities, but apart from that no one was there to point out that sugar might be bad for you.

And that's how we ended up spending 78 percent of our time in senior high baking gooey fudge cake.

WHAT EFFECT DOES SUGAR HAVE ON THE BODY?

We will not delve too deeply into molecular biology in this book, but there are two important things to know if you want to stay healthy and free of inflammation. Those two things are 1) blood sugar, and 2) the blood sugar–lowering hormone *insulin.*

If raw vegetables are yummy for the good bacteria in the colon, then sugar is an absolute delicacy for the nasty bacteria.

Breaking it down, we can say that sugar assists nasty bacteria in encouraging our desire to vacuum up every trace of sugar that comes our way. The more sugar we eat, the louder bad bacteria shouts to our brain that they want more sugar. At this point we need Jane Fonda–like strength and discipline to resist all the candy bowls, sweetened yogurts, office-meeting pastries, sugary drinks, and frequent coffee breaks that are part of our everyday lives.

Unlike fiber, which is processed by the good, protective bacteria in the colon, sugar will head straight into the bloodstream from the small intestine, leaving our army of hungry, good bacteria in the colon in a lurch. Blood sugar levels will spike, which causes the pancreas to begin pumping out more insulin than necessary. When the level of insulin in the body rises, the immune system goes into overdrive, which in turn exhausts the intestinal flora, resulting in inflammation in the body.

Does that mean that the body doesn't need any sugar at all, ever? Not quite. The body needs sugar, but it depends entirely on which area of the intestine it is being absorbed from, what kind of sugar we're talking about, and what types of foods we're getting it from. When common white table sugar ends up in the body, half of it is broken down into what is called *fructose* and the other half into *glucose.* Studies show that it is primarily fructose that is instrumental to poor health. We can summarize it this way: fructose (found in abundance in soft drinks and candy, among other things) is anything but good for us, while glucose (also plentiful in soft drinks and candy, but in vegetables, too) is something we need to ensure good health.

In the right amount, glucose is the body's most important source of energy—not least for the proper working of the brain—so long as you make sure to get it from vegetables and not from sweet rolls. What is important here is how quickly the glucose is processed by the body. Glucose that is absorbed in the small intestine washes over our inner organs and the body like a tsunami, while glucose that is processed by the colon flows like a calm stream in the time it takes the bacteria to break it down.

Leafy greens and other vegetables are good sources of glucose. In spinach, for instance, the level of sugar is low while the level of fiber is high. This is close to being optimal, since the small intestine lacks enzymes to break down the fibers and release the sugar. In contrast to sugar from a cinnamon roll, spinach will continue to make its way all the way down into the colon, unobstructed, where the good bacteria will break it down, and mete out the glucose slowly, which protects the internal organs from receiving more sugar than they can cope with, all at once and at the same time. The body gleans energy from the sugar without a dramatic spike in blood sugar.

The WHO considers that for good health, our total daily intake of energy from sugar should not exceed 5 percent of the total energy intake (this is half of what is officially recommended by the USDA's Dietary Guidelines 2015–2020).

WORLD HEALTH ORGANIZATION POINTS TO SUGAR AS THE GREATEST THREAT TO OUR HEALTH

We still consume far more sugar than we should, despite current scientific research telling us that sugar is detrimental to our health. The WHO (World Health Organization) recommends that women eat no more than 100 calories (25 g or 6 teaspoons of sugar) per day, and men no more than 150 calories (38 g or 9 teaspoons) per day. In America, we eat on average 92 g or 22 teaspoons per day, two to three times the recommended amount. We eat, on average, 150 lb of sugar per person, per year. This is total madness, considering that the WHO points to sugar as the greatest threat to health in the world and the most significant factor in obesity. Research shows that if a child drinks one can of soft drink per day, the likelihood that this child will be overweight later in life is increased by 60 percent.

In America, about 34 percent of all adults have consumed so much sugar that their bodies' natural system for breaking it down is ready to quit. (In Sweden, the number is 15 to 20 percent.) This is called *metabolic syndrome,* which is the precursor to illness, specifically to type 2 diabetes. Simply put, having constantly elevated blood sugar levels eventually leads to a decreased reaction to the insulin pumped out by the body. This in turn leads to a pancreas that needs to produce even more insulin, which brings on a further rise in blood sugar. If this cycle keeps going for too long, the body becomes exhausted and the system for regulating blood sugar is wrecked. When the body's system is upset, the good bacteria in the colon says "thanks, but no thanks." They turn over operations to the Darth Vaders, which we know by now is the primary reason for inflammation and chronic illness.

Excess abdominal fat is an important sign of metabolic syndrome, but even slim people can suffer from metabolic syndrome.

Lina and Mia sit on the pier outside Mia's country house and gaze at the boats making their way into the Swedish island of Marstrand.

– Good grief. This means that almost one in five Swedes is in the danger zone for type 2 diabetes!

– It's even worse when you consider that type 2 diabetes increases our risk of getting sick from an awful number of other illnesses most of us are terrified of.

– Uh-oh, this is bringing on an anxiety attack.

– But, but . . . can you explain to me why I feel like a boring and bad parent when I don't allow my children to eat candy and drink sodas?

– Well, it is weird. It's as if we need to apologize and make up a good excuse for wanting to avoid eating sugar.

Lina ties her hair in a topknot, removes her swim wrap, and prepares to get into the water for a swim.

– When I was at the kindergarten's end-of-term celebration last week, it was the first time I didn't want to throw myself at the plates of cookies and cakes.

– God, that's a wonderful feeling.

– Yeah, but then a mom came up to me and said I should indulge and have a roll. That comment made me feel so stupid and goody-two-shoes that I immediately gorged on three cookies just to prove to her that I was normal.

– I've been in that situation, too.
– Weird, when we've just started to understand how the body works . . .
– That's true . . .
Lina adjusts the floaties on her arms and jumps into the mirror like sea.

OUR OVERALL INTAKE OF SUGAR

Relax, enjoying a piece of candy from time to time never hurt anyone, right? True enough, a bit of chocolate isn't a big deal. The problem is it rarely ends up being a few pieces now and then—studies show that most of us indulge in treats such as candy, chocolates, pastries, and sodas every day. There are frequent coffee breaks, cozy Friday nights, Saturday parties, Sunday picnics, and holidays, such as Easter, Thanksgiving, and Christmas. Add to this the fact that the sizes of buns and bags of candy are three times the size they were back in the 1980s, and that the food industry adds sugar to more than 75 percent of all processed food. Yep, you read that right: most processed food in today's grocery stores contain added sugar, and we're not just talking about the obviously sweet items like breakfast cereals, yogurts, and juices. It's also in ham, many different types of bread, and drinks.

While we're on the subject, why don't we take at closer look at bread for a second? Turn over a packet of any brand of bread and home in on the nutrition label. First, let's look for "Carbohydrates" in the table, and then go down the line. Typically, there's a sub-line, "Sugars," that tells us how much sugar, both naturally occurring and added, is in the product. To find out if there is any added sugar in the product, locate the "Ingredients" list further down the table and look for words like "high-fructose corn syrup," "fructose," "corn syrup," "honey," "molasses," "dextrose," "cane sugar," "fruit juice concentrate," "glucose," "sucrose," "maltose," "lactose," "agave nectar," etc. If you are holding in your hands a popular brand of bread, check to see if any of these words are present, which indicate that the product has added sugars.

Type 2 diabetes was formerly known as adult-onset diabetes, but now in the US type 2 diabetes is prevalent even among children.

We'll say it again: Our bodies can handle us enjoying an occasional chocolate éclair, but today's excessive consumption of sugar clearly contributes to impaired intestinal flora, inflammation, and many other health-related problems. It's enough to make us start looking at sugar more as a spice rather than as a major ingredient in our food. Sugar should not be consumed in large quantities, nor should it be consumed daily. Many scientific studies involving human and animal test subjects have demonstrated that sugar is as satisfying and addictive as alcohol and cocaine—if not more so—and yet still we give it to our children just about every day.

According to federal dietary recommendations, children should not get more than 10 percent of their daily calories from added sugar. This number is exceeded by many by the time they leave the breakfast table.

OUR SENSES NEED A SUGAR DETOX

Since we eat way too much sugar, which isn't just bad for our intestinal flora but is also very addictive, it might be a good idea to send our senses off on a sugar detox. Research shows that it takes about one month for the body to break a sugar habit, which means you need four weeks' time to 1) abstain from eating sugar entirely, and 2) not replace it with any other types of sweetener, since that would keep triggering cravings for sugar. You should steel yourself for a rough start, but after only a few days your cravings will simmer down. And whenever you taste something sugary after that, you'll notice that your tolerance for sweetness will have changed. After a sugar detox, you'll find that your usual three o'clock treat tastes far too sweet.

If you feel motivated to give it a try, turn to page 136 for help. There, you'll find tips under "Project: Save Your Intestinal Flora." However, sugar *is* a habit, and even if you've carefully cleaned out your fridge, prepared yourself mentally, and have written up to-do lists, cravings can kick in at any time with surprising intensity. You'll need to have 1) a backup plan, and 2) a Banana Milkshake with Berry Swirl close at hand. Please, turn the page.

BANANA MILKSHAKE WITH BERRY SWIRL

(makes 2 glasses)

$^4/_5$ cup (200 ml) mixed summer berries

4 tbsp chia seeds

$^2/_5$ cup (100 ml) water

$^4/_5$ tsp (4 ml) vanilla powder, divided

2 cups (500 ml) milk of your choice

2 small green bananas

This recipe has everything two sweet-toothed children (and their parents) could wish for: four different types of berries, spiced vanilla, and yummy banana.

Defrost the berries if they are frozen, and blend them with chia seeds, water, and half of the vanilla powder. Blend the milk, bananas, and remaining vanilla powder separately in another container. Divide the chia seed mixture into two glasses, and add in the banana milk. Stir—think "swirl." Call someone who you believe deserves a milkshake. What—no one's home? It's your lucky day, then: they're both for you.

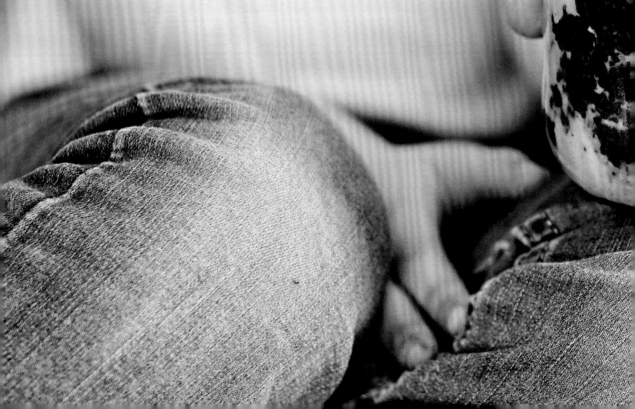

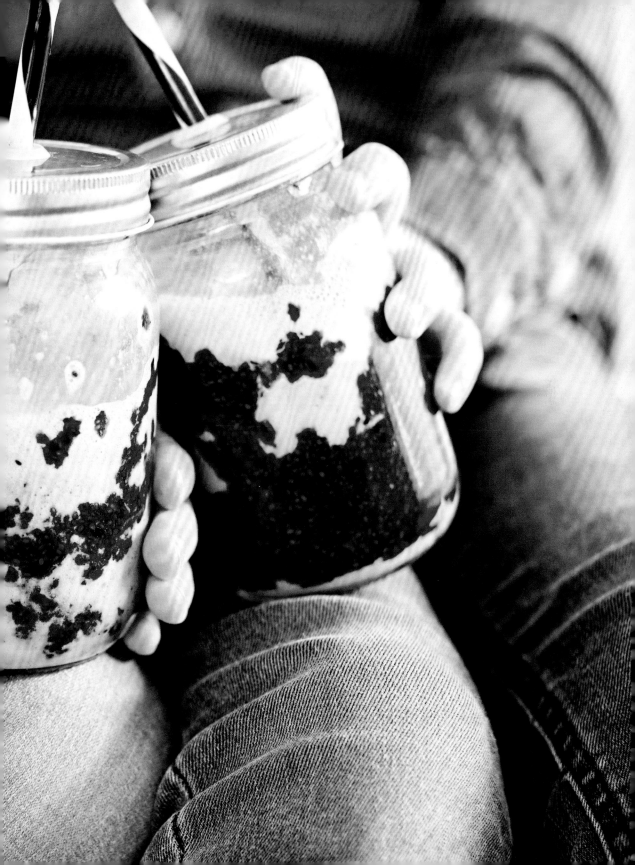

PROJECT SUGAR DETOX—BACKUP PLAN

Studies show that the following activities can help when sugar cravings strike:

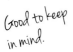

Good to keep in mind.

1 Drink a cup of green tea (this will stabilize your blood sugar).
2 Brush your teeth.
3 Make a green smoothie or eat some grapefruit (green vegetables and citrus fruits are effective at quashing sugar cravings).
4 Get out and move.
5 Call a friend and ask her or him to give you a pep talk to remind you why you should not eat sugar.

LIFE AFTER A SUGAR DETOX

Today, one in ten American children suffer from a condition called fatty liver disease—formerly only seen in alcoholics.

We plowed through pretty much all available pregnancy literature when we were expecting. Once in the delivery room, we knew everything—what type of pain relief we needed, how we wanted to give birth, and that we did not care to eat the placenta. However, what we didn't know was how life was going to turn out *after* the delivery. Suddenly, there we were, each of us with a baby in our arms, with no clue how to handle our new reality. Why hadn't anyone prepared us for all the things that were going to happen after giving birth? After all, this is when things get hard.

We feel that the same applies to detoxing from sugar. Giving up sweets for a certain amount of time is one thing, but what do you do once the detox period is over?

At first, we thought that our new life after the detox would never be the same, but we soon discovered to our great delight that we could still enjoy treats every day. The best source of sweetness is in fruit and berries (both fresh and dried), since their sugar is different from white table sugar. Fruit sugar contains antioxidants and fiber, which help slow the sugar's absorption into the bloodstream. However, we need to raise a tiny red flag here because this doesn't mean you can pig out on baked goods, even if they're made with honey instead of table sugar. Though we stopped using white sugar, we continued to bake many treats using dried figs, apricots, and dates as sweeteners instead, and while they were much better for our intestinal flora, they unfortunately kept triggering our sweet cravings. It wasn't until we cooled things off—even with alternative sweetening agents— that we managed to control our sweet tooth more effectively for the first time.

Therefore, the following applies in the ideal world:
1 Save those date truffles for special occasions.
2 Add flavor with anti-inflammatory spices such as cardamom, cocoa, and cinnamon, which all have the nifty ability to lower blood sugar.
3 Add in some coconut oil, since fat also keeps blood sugar from rising too much (more on this later on).

To satisfy your senses, you can try to focus on treats that won't fire up inflammation but provide healthy nutrients instead. You'll find lots of them here:
1 Frozen green banana on a stick, dipped in melted dark chocolate (85 percent cocoa or higher)
2 Mixed natural nuts and coconut flakes
3 Seed crackers
4 Kale chips
5 Smoothies made with avocados and berries
6 Ice cream made with frozen berries, frozen sliced banana, coconut cream, and anti-inflammatory spices
7 Frozen grapes

You can enjoy many of the snacks listed above on a daily basis. A coffee break with raspberries, coconut flakes, cinnamon, and cardamom contains fiber, antioxidants, and anti-inflammatory spices, which won't just make homework easier but will also boost intestinal flora. And those banana muffins on the following page— don't even get us started! Their only sweeteners are three green bananas, which allows even those of you who are diabetic to enjoy them without your insulin going nuts. We could almost say it'd be crazy to eat just one, knowing how many good fats and anti-inflammatory ingredients they contain, such as coconut oil, green bananas, walnuts, cinnamon, and lingonberries.

Avoid sweeteners, at least during your period of sugar detox, since they only bring on sugar cravings.

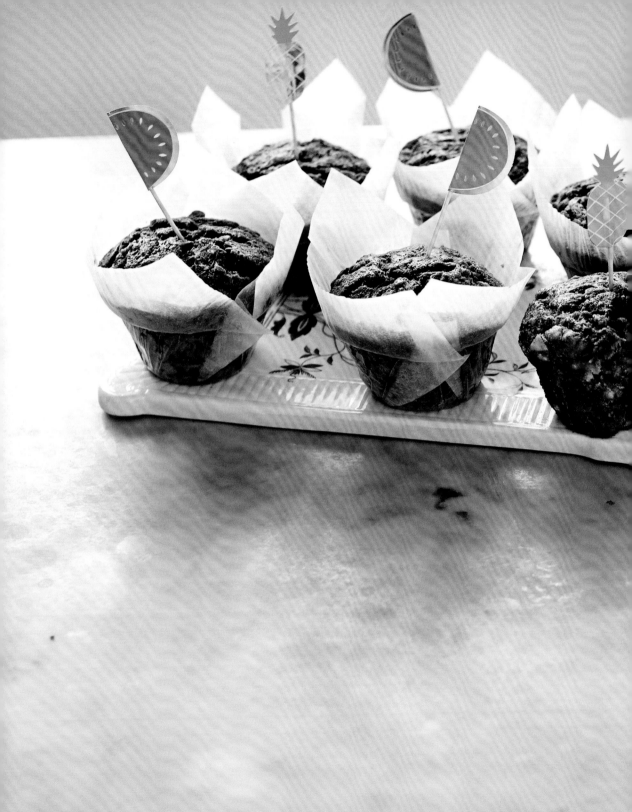

BLOOD SUGAR–FRIENDLY BANANA MUFFINS

(so sorry, only makes 8)

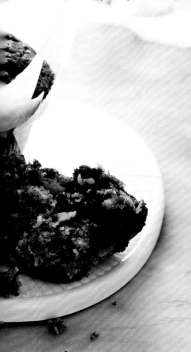

²/₅ cup (100 ml) sorghum flour

¹/₅ tsp (1 ml) baking soda

1 tbsp (15 ml) ground cinnamon

1 tsp (5 ml) vanilla powder

¹/₅ tsp (1 ml) sea salt

2 large eggs

²/₅ cup (100 ml) coconut oil

⁴/₅ cup (200 ml) mashed bananas (2–3 bananas)

²/₅ cup (100 ml) lingonberries (or cranberries)

²/₅ cup (100 ml) walnuts, coarsely chopped

We often bring these muffins along on our picnics. It's not quite clear if we organize outings to have an excuse to bake banana muffins, or if we bake banana muffins because we want to have a picnic. Whatever the case may be, they regularly go into the oven and then with us on our jaunts.

Preheat the oven to at most 212°F (100°C). Mix flour, baking soda, cinnamon, vanilla, and sea salt in a bowl and set aside. Whisk together the eggs and the oil, and pour over the dry ingredients. Add the mashed bananas, lingonberries, and walnuts to the batter. Pour the batter into 8 muffin tins and bake about 1 hour. (Use a toothpick to check for doneness.) Remove from the oven and let cool (if you can stand the wait).

GREEN BANANAS

When Mia was in kindergarten, she always carried a green banana in her backpack whenever she went on picnics with her class. The banana had to be perfectly green, very rough in texture, and stick to the roof of her mouth like glue; if it didn't fulfill those requirements she didn't want it. The other kids watched her skeptically as she fought to remove the peel from the unripe fruit, but Mia persevered. To this day, she still thinks ripe bananas are one of the grossest things ever.

But here is where she gets satisfaction: Professor Stig explained that this is probably an inherent, ancestral instinct. When good-for-you vegetable fibers ripen, they morph into unhealthy sugar, a typical example being the banana. It is chock-full of fibers at the onset, but as it ripens it turns into simple sugars.

Green bananas, in contrast to their yellow (or half-rotten, per Stig) counterparts, are rich in pectin, which is paradise for intestinal flora. Our ancestors consumed greens and plants long before they were ripe, as do wild apes. In addition to fiber, bananas are rich in vitamins and minerals. Remember to choose organic bananas when shopping, because grocery store bananas are, sadly, heavily treated with pesticides. And don't look dubiously at a kid on the bus who tries to nosh on a green banana.

It is an inherent, ancestral instinct, just so you know.

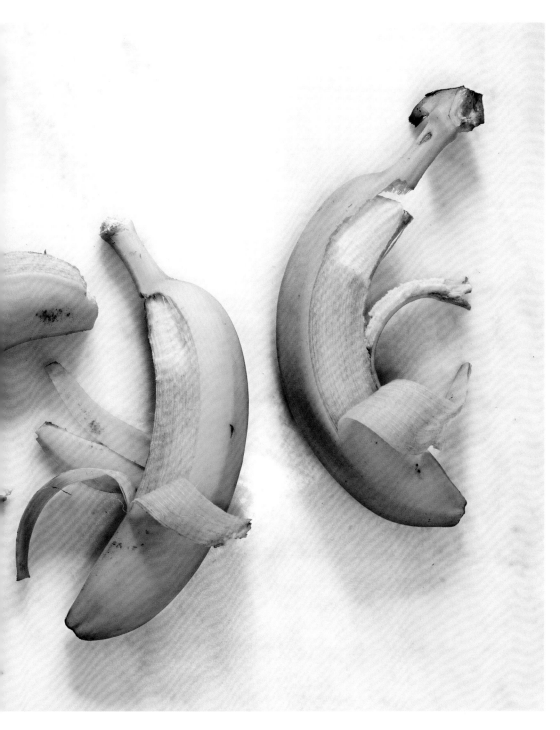

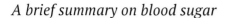

A brief summary on blood sugar

FIVE SWEET TIPS FOR GOOD INTESTINAL FLORA

01. Start by quitting soda and all sweetened drinks.
Sorry, but liquid sugar is one of the very worst types of sweeteners out there.

02. Do you like to bake? Great! You can start experimenting with these recipes. Test one without using white sugar, just for the heck of it. Whaddya say?

03. Freeze some green bananas so you can make your own ice cream in no time.

04. Freeze organic grapes, so you always have a popsicle handy.

05. Craving fruit salad? Cram in lots of berries and preferably an acidic fruit, such as grapefruit, and go ahead and season it with cinnamon, cardamom, cocoa, and other anti-inflammatory goodies.

BECOME A NUTRIENT HUNTER

(and say goodbye to the morning-after belly)

Congratulations, you have just been prescribed spaghetti and meat sauce. Without spaghetti, naturally. And wouldn't you know it, with no meat sauce, either. Aside from the fact that your entire family will love this dish, it's also anti-inflammatory (surprise, surprise) and full of green wonders. Contrary to regular pasta, which is quickly absorbed by the small intestine and converted to sugar in the body, this vegetable pasta travels effortlessly all the way down to the good bacteria in the colon. You do recall, don't you? The difference in whether you're feeding Luke or Darth lies in where the food is absorbed—early in the small intestine or a little later, in the colon. Sugary foods are absorbed quickly in the small intestine, which causes an unnecessary elevation of blood sugar. This is exactly what this chapter is going to be about—the difference between nutrient-rich food that boosts the intestinal flora and nutrient-poor stomach fillers.

OUR SUGAR CV (PART 2)

– *Would you like some bread?*

Our waiter places a large basket of bread just under the tip of Lina's nose. She happily grabs two slices of bread, pours some olive oil on the plate, and sops the bread in the oil.

– *I don't really eat bread . . .*

The waiter looks at her, puzzled.

– *Pardon me?*

Lina puts a piece of bread in her mouth and starts chewing.

– *Well, I used to live on bread. I always had an egg sandwich with fish roe spread for breakfast, and then a few more slices of bread at lunch. Around 4 p.m. I used to snack on a few crispbreads, and when I got home at the end of the day I had slices of toast for dinner. I used to eat a boatload of spaghetti, too. And macaroni. And rice. I had no idea that this was not good for my intestinal flora.*

Lina mops another chunk of bread in the oil until every drop of it is absorbed. She puts it in her mouth.

– *But then I realized that this kind of food provides no nutrition. Stig calls it "sugar-simulating" food because it behaves exactly like sugar when you eat it. I didn't understand any of this at the beginning. I had no idea that rice and pasta and pizza and that kind of stuff acted like sugar in the blood. I thought only table sugar was bad. So I began by limiting the amount of bread I ate. I haven't cut it out completely—that would be too hard—but sometimes you find yourself in situations where it's impossible to say no. And when my mo—*

(By now the waiter has left our table, but you can already guess whether Lina misses bread or not.)

BAD NEWS

We don't want to be a pair of wet blankets here, but there is something we have to say. As soon as we thought we had completed the sugar detox and begun abiding by our intestinal flora's rules, Professor Stig placed pictures of a baguette, a bag of sugar, and a Snickers bar on the table and asked us which item we thought would elevate our blood sugar the most.

Naturally, we knew this was a trick question. But when Stig told us *the baguette* was the biggest villain, we had some trouble wrapping our minds around it. Here we thought we had just kicked our sugar addiction to the curb, and then we're informed that the sandwich we just had for breakfast dissolves into large amounts of sugar, which is pumped out into the body way too quickly. After taking a look at what we had eaten over the past week, we realized that we literally live on what Stig calls sugar-simulating food.

Wait, what? What do you mean by "sugar-simulating food"? Common to all sugar-simulating food is having a high glycemic Index (GI) and low fiber, antioxidant, vitamin, and mineral content. In other words, they're classic stomach fillers. Sadly, sugar-simulating food is comprised of all those tasty things that many of us eat too much: bread, pasta, pizza, and rice. Characteristic to sugar-simulating food is 1) a lack of nutrients, and 2) having the same effect on blood sugar as everyday table sugar. Sugar-stimulating foods are also readily absorbed by the small intestine; they raise blood sugar, leave our good bacteria in a lurch, and induce inflammation. The body makes no distinction whatsoever between the sugar in a bar of chocolate, a plate of spaghetti, or a crusty bread roll with cheese. This is a huge disappointment to Lina and Mia, as well as to the majority of the population.

Sugar-simulating food contains large amounts of glucose; the good news is that it doesn't have any fructose. It doesn't really matter if you understood the minute distinctions between fructose and glucose in the last chapter or not, so long as you remember that everyone needs a bit of glucose in their diet; it is fructose that should be avoided as much as possible. It's pretty simple: there are foods that provide the body with glucose in a slow and orderly fashion (like spinach), and there is food that overwhelms the body with large surges of glucose (sugar-simulating foods with a high GI). As for the GI? Since glucose goes hand in hand with the glycemic index, we may as well go over the basics right now.

GLYCEMIC INDEX AND NUTRITION

Sugar-simulating foods contain large amounts of carbohydrates, which break down into the type of sugar called glucose in the body. Blood sugar levels spike rapidly if the body receives a large quantity of glucose over a short period of time; by now we know that high blood sugar leads to inflammation in the body. How quickly blood sugar rises and how high it rises depends on the carbohydrate's *glycemic index* (GI). GI is a measurement that shows how quickly 50 g (1.76 oz) of carbohydrate of a certain food causes blood sugar to rise. Add also to this equation the factor that different types of food contain different amounts of carbohydrate. Consuming 50 g (1.76 oz) of carbohydrate is not a problem if all you eat is sugar-simulating food, such as bread, pasta, rice, or boiled potatoes, since they are 20–40 percent carbohydrate. In order to reach that same amount of carbohydrate by eating nothing but raw carrots, you'll have to work a little harder.

When we eat sugar-simulating food like a baguette or macaroni, the body starts to pump out a lot of extra insulin to lower our blood sugar. As the baguette and the macaroni are already absorbed in the small intestine, Luke's army is deprived of food, and this, along with elevated blood sugar, leads to inflammation.

When the body's defense system is disrupted and unable to burn off all the sugar, the body is also forced to store this excess sugar in the fat cells. Consequently, blood sugar takes a nosedive, and an hour later you're hungry again and craving something sweet, which is a pity when you remember that you've only just eaten.

You could say that the more sugar-simulating food we eat, the hungrier we become. Even though we eat and eat until we're stuffed to the gills, we're soon hungry again, and keeping that

SCIENCE FOR YOU

The glycemic index (GI) is used to measure the effect 50 g (1.76 oz) of food has on rising levels of blood sugar. Foods with a high GI elevate blood sugar the most.

insulin is the body's most efficient fat storing hormone, it's not hard to imagine what happens when it is allowed to roam at will in our bloodstream. In that way, sugar-simulating food, like sugar, is highly addictive, and the more we consume it, the more of it we want. The exact opposite happens when we eat raw and unprocessed food: not only does it lead to stable blood sugar levels, which makes us feel full longer, but the breakdown of raw vegetables in the colon doesn't begin until after about one and a half hours, and it takes about five hours to complete.

Mia looks up from the Downward Dog pose.
– (Whispers) So, it's really the total opposite of what many people believe.
Lina looks at her.
– (whispers) What?
– (whispers) Yeah, don't you remember how you felt after that big plate of spaghetti carbonara at lunch? First you were so stuffed that you felt like you were dying and that you had to lie down on the sofa to start writing your will, but then two hours later you were feeling snack-y again, and craving a sweet roll.
Mia changes into the Warrior pose, and Lina follows.
– (whispers) Well, yes, now that you mention it . . .
– (whispers) Yeah, and then you compare that to how you feel after drinking half a quart of green smoothie for lunch. That will carry us for at least five hours, no problem.
– (whispers) Yeah, that's true.
The yoga teacher frowns in their direction.

Today, many people are scared of carbohydrates and tar them all with the same brush, when in fact a large daily intake of food with *low carb concentration* is healthy, contributing to rich intestinal flora and a strong immune system. Thus, not all carbohydrates act like sugar-simulating food, which have a high concentration of carbs, in addition to low nutrient and fiber content. Research shows a strong positive link between consumption of vegetable-based carbohydrates and good health. Vegetables not only have a low concentration of carbohydrates, they are also rich in fiber, and because the carbohydrates are enclosed in fiber, the food will

SCIENCE FOR YOU

An important reason to stay away from sugar-simulating food is that it leads to spikes in blood sugar, weak intestinal flora, and inflammation.

SPAGHETTI AND MEAT SAUCE—MINUS SPAGHETTI AND MEAT SAUCE

(this makes a lot)

Do you have whiny kids? Feel free to switch the vegetable pasta to bean noodles, for example. Use the same spices you add to your usual meat sauce, or mix in some of your meat sauce with our vegetarian version, gradually decreasing the amount meat and increasing the amount of lentils. All roads lead to Rome, right?

$^3/_5$ cup (150 ml) Beluga lentils

1 tbsp vegetarian stock powder

1 garlic clove, peeled and crushed

1 yellow onion, peeled and sliced

$^4/_5$ cup (200 ml) water

1 lb (500 g) crushed tomatoes

2 handfuls baby spinach

1 carrot, peeled and grated

Salt and freshly ground black pepper

2 zucchini

Fresh oregano

Bring the lentils, stock powder, garlic, and onion to a boil in the water. Add the crushed tomatoes when the water has been absorbed. Mix everything with the spinach and grated carrot. Salt and pepper to taste. Grate the zucchini with a mandolin, cheese slicer, or spiralizer. Top with the sauce and serve with sprinkles of anti-inflammatory oregano.

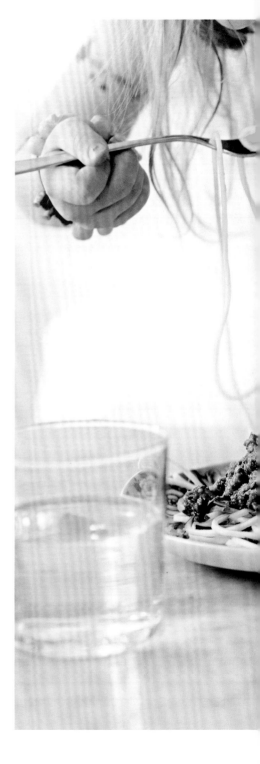

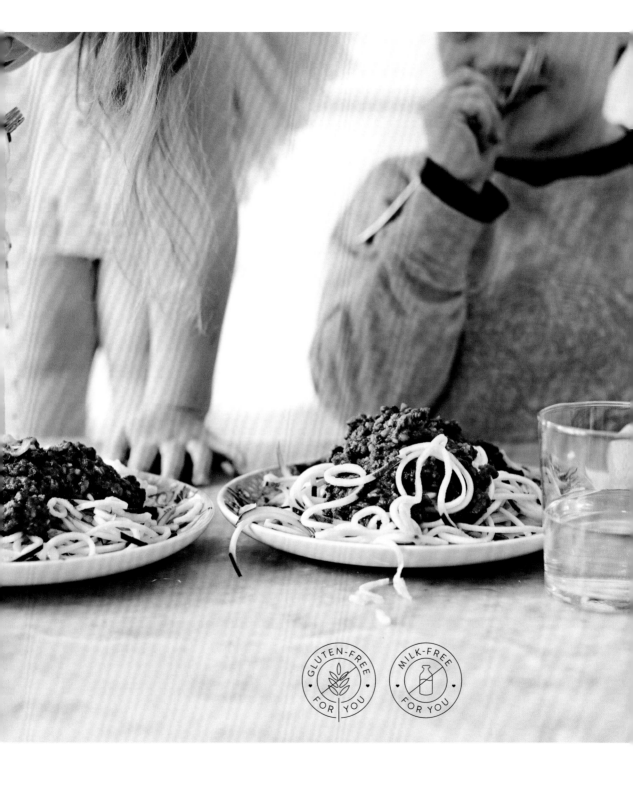

Fig. #3

GLYCEMIC INDEX

We've compiled some good and healthy ingredients that
have low to lower average GI (<55) below:

Black-eyed peas	Buckwheat groats
Kidney beans	Sourdough bread (rye flour)
Mung beans	Unsweetened muesli
Black beans	Apples
Cashews	Barley, whole and cooked
Green and red lentils	Dark chocolate >60 percent cocoa
Chickpeas	Plain yogurt
Green peas	Soba noodles
Grapefruit	Carrots (raw)
Strawberries	Pecans
Potatoes (cooked and cooled)	Mushrooms
Banana (green)	Lemon

Friday treats →

reach all the way down to the colon where it becomes fuel for our good bacteria. The glucose that is now available in the colon is released slowly and in a controlled fashion into the body, and will thus not have a negative effect on blood sugar. As easy as it is to reach 50 g (1.76 oz) of carbohydrates by eating pasta or pizza, it's hard to do so when you're filling up on mushrooms or carrots, since they're only 2–7 percent carbohydrates. This means that even if you eat a carrot, which in and of itself has a high GI, it won't raise your blood sugar by much because it contains so few carbohydrates.

If you plan to follow a strict GI diet, it's important to keep a close eye on the entire meal's GI and not just the raw ingredients. We usually refer to something called *insulin sensitivity,* which is simply the body's ability to handle the large release of insulin that high-carb foods will cause. It's good to aim for high insulin sensitivity, which means that the body only needs to pump out a small amount of insulin to lower blood sugar. Happily, there are many foods that will increase your insulin sensitivity. Food containing water-soluble fibers, magnesium-rich food, healthy fats, fish, fermented food, red wine (!), and foods with low pH = excellent.

At the starting point of our pilgrim's journey towards an anti-inflammatory life, we kept skipping all the information about GI. We had heard and read about it, of course, but almost always in the context of someone's huge weight loss, as in "Larry ate no carbs and dropped 80 lb. He says he owes it all to the GI method." We were interested in food primarily from a health standpoint, so we dismissed the GI as just another weight loss plan. Today, a few years, many diagrams, scientific research reports, discussions, interviews, and books later, we understand that GI is far more than that. GI is a key ingredient in good health and has helped many people all over the world combat obesity, type 2 diabetes, and metabolic syndrome, all without the use of medication. Learning the basics of how food affects blood sugar should be compulsory education.

Fat lowers a meal's total glycemic index (GI).

We may sound as though we're terribly strict adherents to GI, but that isn't the case. However, we do eat foods with low GI first, because there is a clear correlation between low GI and high nutrient density, in the same way there is a link between high GI and low nutrient density.

We normally consider ourselves nutrient hunters. If you seek out a nutrient-rich diet, many foods with high GI automatically fall by the wayside because they are nutrient-poor. That doesn't mean you can stick an equal sign between low GI and healthy; and there are foods with low GI that don't contain any nutrition whatsoever. Fructose, for example, which we talked about earlier, is something we should avoid eating. Inversely, fruit that often has a high GI can at the same time contain tons of fiber and antioxidants, both of which our good bacteria loves.

Fruit is a bit problematic because it can affect blood sugar if eaten in large quantities. Be that as it may, we can't agree that an excess consumption of fruit in the Western world is most likely our main problem. Rather, the trouble is that we eat far too few fruits and vegetables, and all research points to a positive correlation between a hearty fruit habit and good health. However, those of you who enjoy lots of fruit on a daily basis might want to consider swapping some fruit for some vegetables, or choose sour and unripe fruits that contain more fiber and less sugar. We try to think along the lines of the advice from the last chapter about the date truffles—we'd rather eat a cookie sweetened with dates any time over a cookie made with white sugar, but we're also conscious that we still shouldn't overdo it.

WHY DO PEOPLE EAT SO MUCH SUGAR-SIMULATING FOOD?

At first, we had some trouble believing that most of the food we ate every day caused inflammation. We couldn't stop wondering how things could have taken such a bad turn. Out of all the wonderful foods we could pick from, most of our meals consisted of sugar-simulating food. Why was that? Was it even true? Was it indeed the case that the food we, and everyone we know, lives off, is as damaging and can lead to as many problems as scientists predict?

Okay, here we go:

We are both nearing our forties. Sure, we look twenty-five by candlelight. In other words, we were born in the 1970s, and so we grew up in Sweden at a time when the common man had no idea what sugar-simulating food was. This was during the era when the Food Administration recommended that we consume six to eight slices of bread (a sugar-simulating food) per day, and our home economic teachers happily waved the "Plate Diet Model" around (which was made up of mostly sugar-simulating foods).

According to this plate model, a meal should consist of 40 percent *carbohydrates*, 40 percent *fiber*, and 20 percent *protein*. As we know now, broccoli and red cabbage are good carbs, but for some reason the Food Administration opted to put all vegetables in the "fiber" category. This means that the plate's 40 percent carbohydrates go mostly to sugar-simulating foods such as pasta, bread, rice, and cooked potatoes (we will look more in-depth at potatoes later, so hold that thought). We grew up with a food model in which almost *half* of our meal consisted of sugar-simulating food—food that is nutrient-poor but rich in "sugar," food that leads to inflammation and chronic disease. It's not surprising we were confused.

Another reason why sugar-simulating food is such a large part of our diet today could be that we're so used to eating the least healthy part of, say, seeds and grains, while giving the good-for-you parts (the hull and germ) to livestock. Take wheat, for example. Wheat can be roughly separated into three parts: the hull, germ, and flour. The flour consists only of empty calories while the bran (hull) and germ are the healthy parts. Strangely enough, ours is a food culture in which we consume the flour (the empty calories) and leave the hull and bran to the pigs to aid their digestion, as well as to farmed minks to give them glossy coats. If we had done the opposite and concentrated on the germ and hull, our food would have behaved completely differently in our body.

A third reason why we eat so much sugar-simulating food is because a lot of food has been refined (heated, for instance), which transforms fiber to sugar. Before raw ingredients are processed by food manufacturers (or in-home in the kitchen), glucose is encased in fibers to enable it to go all the way down into the colon, where it is released to be used by good bacteria for energy, which has a positive effect on the body and will not spike blood sugar. But if raw ingredients are manipulated to become sugar-simulating products before we ingest them, glucose is released as soon as it hits the small intestine and results in quick energy and a spike in blood sugar, which can damage the body's organs in the long run.

Elevated blood sugar and elevated insulin levels are important factors in type 2 diabetes, which in turn increases the risk of developing many other chronic diseases.

SO WE'RE NOT EVEN ALLOWED TO EAT POTATOES, THEN?

The hawk-eyed among us will have noted that America's (and Sweden's) national carb, the potato, belongs in the sugar-simulating group. We don't mean to scare you, so we'll set your mind at ease by telling you that this only applies to warm potatoes. Potatoes contain a fiber called *resistant starch,* which is one of the most beneficial substances for our good bacteria. Resistant starch is one of the principal sources of the short-chain fatty acids that line the intestine and reduce inflammation. One hundred percent of the resistant starch reaches all the way down into the colon—studies have shown that daily consumption of 0.5–1 oz (15–30 g) of resistant starch strongly protects against metabolic syndrome (you know, the pre-diabetic stage that precedes type 2 diabetes we talked about in the last chapter). Better still, resistant starch is known to fight obesity. It's no exaggeration to proclaim resistant starch a mighty fine fiber.

There's one tiny catch, however: resistant starch turns into sugar when potatoes are cooked. But you can easily solve this problem by letting the potato—and other root vegetables—cool down before you eat them. *Sorry, did you say* cool down*?* That's right. When root vegetables are heated, the fibers disappear and become sugar, but if you let them cool a bit after cooking, they'll revert to being fibers again and travel all the way down to our friends in the colon. A more elegant term for this phenomenon is "recrystallization." Once you've cooked and cooled the tubers, you can actually reheat them without the fibers turning back into sugar. It's as if we had a bit of magic happening here.

WHAT ON EARTH ARE WE GOING TO EAT?

Decreasing the consumption of sugar-simulating foods might be considered by many as one of the most difficult things to do, at least in the beginning, especially since those foods are typically the foundation of our daily diet. When we decided to cut out most of the food we ate in one day, we were almost ready to throw in the towel. First white sugar, and now *this*? Our heads spun. Would we ever be allowed to enjoy bread at breakfast again? What about pasta, which is so tasty and filling; how could anyone even think of trading that in for zucchini? Cold, cooked potatoes—you're joking, right? So what? We had to rethink everything because of our intestinal flora.

In the ideal world, this would be happening:
1 Eat as many whole foods as possible, because unprocessed food usually has a lower GI.
2 You don't have to remove something just because its GI is higher—remember to check its nutrient density.
3 Fats and fibers lower the GI of the entire meal.

!!!

How about in the physical, real world? Well, we won't let ourselves go blind poring over lists. Not to disparage GI tables, but what works best for us is to think about what we can give to the body, not about what we need to remove from it. We have discovered that if you think about food as fuel for the body and make sure to replenish it with as many nutrients as possible each day, in the end there is no room left over for stomach "fillers."

Why not have a trial run by making the potato salad on the next page? Place it on a pretty plate and eat until you're satiated. How do you feel? How does your body feel? Do you crave pasta? Bread? Rice?

We didn't think so.

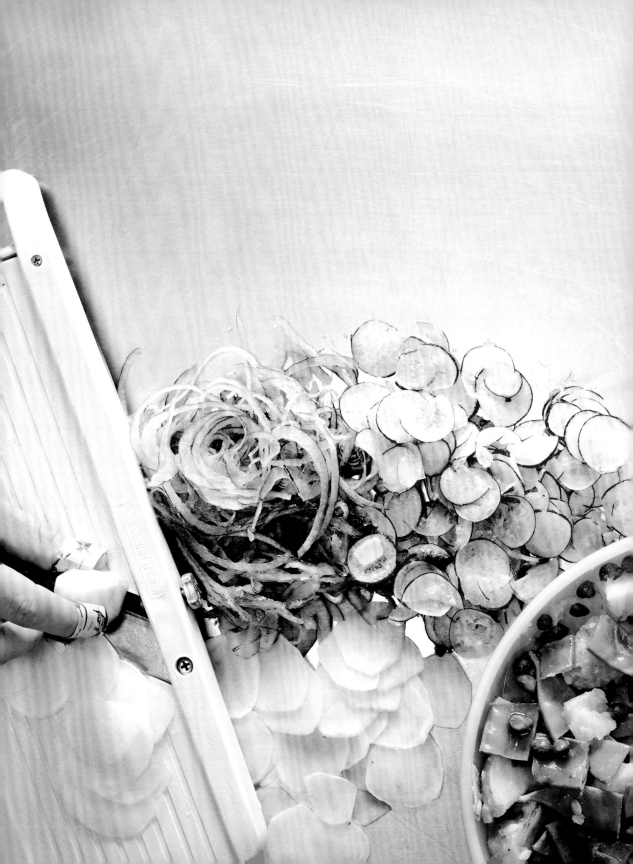

COLD POTATO SALAD THAT WILL TRAVEL ALL THE WAY DOWN TO FEED YOUR INTESTINAL FLORA

(enough for you and 3 hungry pals)

We eat this cold and fiber-rich potato salad regularly—especially in the summer—and often with a piece of fish. Use a mandolin or a cheese slicer, and keep an economy pack of Band-Aids nearby.

Start by boiling the potatoes. Cut them into smaller chunks. Cut up the sugar snap peas and finely slice the radishes, red onion, and the Jerusalem artichokes.

Add the vegetables to the chunks of potato and parsley. Whisk the olive oil, vinegar, mustard, capers, salt, and pepper together in a bowl to make a dressing. Mix everything together and let it sit awhile before you holler that food is ready.

Vegetables

1½ lb (250 g) potatoes

3½ oz (100 g) sugar snap peas

1 bunch radishes

½ red onion, peeled

4 Jerusalem artichokes

2 tbsp finely chopped parsley

French vinaigrette

⅕ cup (50 ml) olive oil

1 tbsp red wine vinegar

1 tsp Dijon mustard

1 tbsp finely chopped capers

Salt and freshly ground black pepper

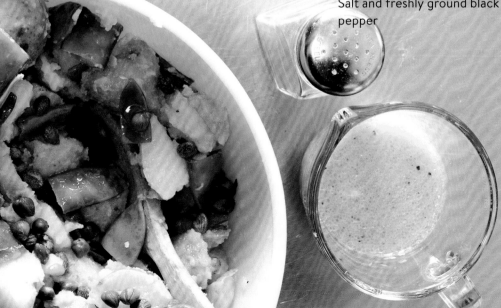

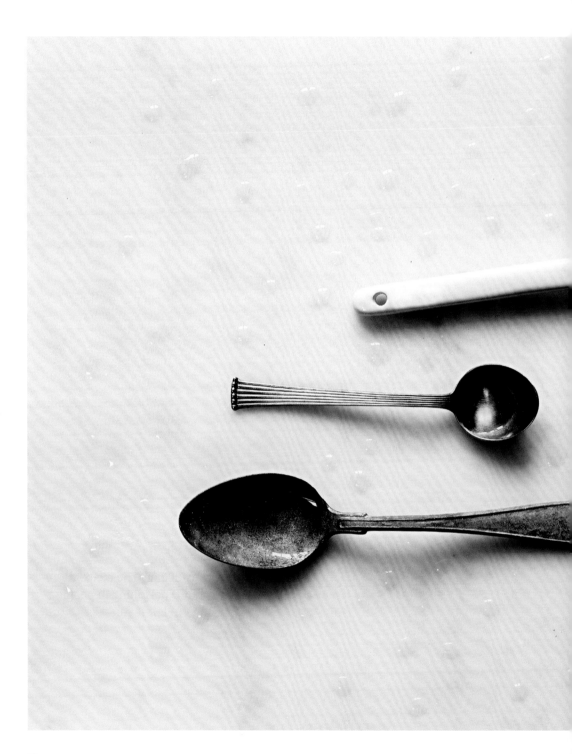

VITAMIN D

There are many advantages to living in Sweden, for us. Needing to carry a flashlight and use a reflective jacket six months out of the year when you want to be outside is not one of them.

We have such little access to sunlight in northern Europe during the cold half of the year that we are hardly able to make any vitamin D (fortunately, if you live in America, you will be exposed to more sunlight). If we don't take vitamin D in supplements, we need to depend on the amount we can stockpile in summer. Professor Stig taught us that vitamin D's half-life is 6 weeks, which means you lose half of your stashed vitamin D every six weeks. If you don't take a vacation in a sunny place in the fall, your vitamin D stores will be empty just in time for the Christmas break. The lack of vitamin D reaches its nadir in March and April, which is when most chronic conditions worsen. Rates of depression peak a few months beforehand.

Vitamin D strengthens the immune system and decreases inflammation in the body, keeping you healthy and alert. We have made it a habit to always take vitamin D supplements. The recommended dose of vitamin D is 15 micrograms or 600 IU (IU = International Units) per day for children and adults; if you're seventy-five or over you should double the daily dose to 20 micrograms/800 IU. The media has reported on cases of vitamin D poisoning in people who have taken too much of it, but if you stick to the recommended amounts, there's no risk of toxicity.

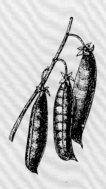

A FEW THINGS ON THE IMPORTANCE OF CHOOSING ORGANIC PRODUCE

Do you think it's expensive to fill an entire shopping cart with organic produce? Then start by buying just a few vegetables that will make a difference in our environment and for us humans. In the United States, researchers tested and ranked the chemical content of fifty-three different fruits and vegetables, and the results are collected in two nifty lists called The Dirty Dozen and The Clean Fifteen. The Dirty Dozen consists of the vegetables and fruit that contain the highest levels of chemicals—items that you should always seek out in their organic state—and the Clean Fifteen lists the fruit and vegetables with the lowest levels of chemicals, meaning you can buy them conventionally grown at the grocery store (but you should avoid them anyway, in solidarity with the field workers).

We understand that many believe they simply can't afford to buy organic, but think of it this way: it costs nothing to avoid buying the very worst items on the list of chemical-laden produce.

Fig. #4

THE DIRTY DOZEN AND THE CLEAN FIFTEEN

Source: American Environmental Working Group (EWG)

Dirty dozen!	Clean fifteen!
1. Apples	1. Avocado
2. Celery	2. Corn
3. Tomatoes	3. Pineapple
4. Cucumbers	4. Cabbage
5. Grapes	5. Peas
6. Nectarines	6. Onions
7. Peaches	7. Asparagus
8. Potatoes	8. Mangoes
9. Spinach	9. Papaya
10. Strawberries	10. Kiwi
11. Blueberries (farmed)	11. Eggplant
12. Bell Peppers	12. Honeydew melon
	13. Grapefruit
	14. Cantaloupe melon
	15. Cauliflower

Bananas are missing from the list. They are also heavily treated with pesticides.

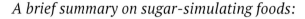

A brief summary on sugar-simulating foods:

FIVE TURBO TIPS FOR INTESTINAL FLORA

01. Start by cleaning out your pantry. A tired cliché, yes, but it works. Throw out or give away the following: pasta, rice, bread, and white flour. Don't cheat. Just get rid of it!

02. Go shopping and buy nutrient-rich alternatives to stomach fillers: quinoa, sorghum flour, mung bean noodles, seeds, nuts, buckwheat, etc.

03. Let root vegetables cool down after cooking them. It may sound a bit boring, but try it and you'll see that when you serve them with warm food, you'll hardly notice the difference.

04. It's a common misconception that meals need to feature some type of grain. A piece of fish and a big salad, instead of a nutrient-poor grain, is just as replenishing. Or a hearty soup. Or a sumptuous stew. You'll be satisfied—we promise.

05. If you can't imagine not having bread, try to bake your own, or at least buy it from a proper, stand-alone bakery instead of picking it up from the grocery store.

GORGE ON VEGETABLES

(to make things more fun for your intestinal flora)

We've now reached the third prescription of the book. And let us guess: this is the first time your prescription mentions lentil soup. If you've been keeping up with our blog you'll know that we like to use magic, and this is one of our best magic tricks. Here we've managed to eat a large amount of raw vegetables, all within a comforting soup. Unlike many other dinners, this one takes nearly five hours to digest. We know it sounds like we're exaggerating, but you will feel fuller eating this vegetable soup than any pasta or rice dish.

By the way, this is the longest chapter in the book because we simply love vegetables more than anything. More than life itself. More than Benicio del Toro.

OUR VEGETABLE CV (CURRICULUM VITAE)

Once upon a time we felt that steak with béarnaise sauce was the ultimate meal. In those days, we'd meet up at our favorite eatery down the block, consume our meat, and silently lick our plates clean without giving a second thought to health, the environment, or other restaurant patrons. Years have passed. We have since married, had children, lost a mom and an aunt to cancer, become hypochondriacs, resigned from our jobs, met Professor Stig, launched a blog, gotten to know a science journalist and a few chief physicians, listened to Johan Rockström, who talked about global warming on his summertime talk-radio show, watched a bunch of documentaries, and along the way decided to start eating a lot of vegetables, and just a little bit of meat, out of interest for our health as well as for our Earth.

It was tough at first because we had always planned our meals starting off with meat, naturally. Lamb chops, filets of beef, or sausage—what was it going to be? What about a side dish: spaghetti, rice, or macaroni? Vegetables always seemed to come up last, if they came up at all.

But then it happened, seemingly all by itself. We made the ultimate discovery that you can feel satisfied on vegetable soup, and that you can make wonderfully creamy sauces from soaked cashews. *A sauce from cashews?* This is when our friends began to worry. *What's happening to Mia and Lina? Have they lost their minds?* And while they plotted how to save us from ourselves, we stopped planning which vegetable would go with our choice of meat and instead decided whether we were going to add any meat at all to our vegetables.

Today, we eat according to this plan: lots of vegetables and only a little bit of meat. And we feel so much better and far more alert than ever before. Someone mentioned that, based on what we do and eat, we are considered flexitarians, but we don't think it matters what you call it. We don't call it anything. We don't like to compartmentalize. Can we just stop pigeonholing things? Can't we just do what we enjoy, and eat lots of things that make us feel good, and a few less of things that are not so good for us?

And yes, every day we do spend a bit of time wondering how we can make a really tasty beef stroganoff without beef.

MOST PEOPLE DON'T EAT ENOUGH VEGETABLES

There is quite a lot of conflicting research about food. There are studies showing that meat is good for us, and studies indicating that meat is bad for us. There are studies suggesting that milk contributes to certain illnesses, and studies proving that it inhibits others. There is research showing that coffee is one of the strongest antioxidants out there, but that its processing makes it toxic. As you can see, you could just go crazy.

However, so far we haven't encountered a single scientist who claims that a copious and varied intake of vegetables is anything but great for your health. Now that we've grasped the basics—that vegetables feed our army of good bacteria—things suddenly seem to make sense. Vegetables are, quite simply, full of all the things our good bacteria need: vitamins, minerals, antioxidants, and fiber. They keep blood sugar stable, and many vegetables are also alkaline. For optimal absorption of nutrients in the colon, our food's pH level needs to be slightly alkaline. Bearing in mind that most of what we consume today makes our digestive environment acidic, it's very important that we consume lots of alkaline food. It is noted that vegetables forcefully fight chronic inflammation, and their absence could eventually lead to chronic disease.

Always drizzle some cold-pressed olive oil, rapeseed oil, or flaxseed oil over vegetables. The body requires fat to properly absorb nutrients from vegetables.

Unlike many other types of food, there doesn't seem to be an upper limit at which point the intake of different vegetables becomes dangerous instead of healthy. In contrast, we know for sure that there is a base limit. The USDA's 2015–2020 Dietary Guidelines suggests a daily base amount of 2½–3 cups of vegetables per day , but many researchers feel that we should consume much more—up to about 5 cups of vegetables per day, depending on your weight and activity level. Sadly, the average American eats about 1½–2 cups of veggies a day.

THE VITAL VEGETABLE FIBER

It is commonly believed that only the vitamins, minerals, and antioxidants are the important components of vegetables, but that is far from the whole story. We want to take this opportunity to, once more, make the case for fiber. Did you know that fiber is made up of carbohydrates that the small intestine can't break down? That's the reason why it travels all the way down to the colon, where it becomes ideal nutrition for your good bacteria. Some fiber is called "probiotic"—the meaning of that word is "food for bacteria," which is apt since much of the fiber is just that: super vital nourishment for our good bacteria. The reason is twofold:

1 It's difficult for the body to digest vegetable fiber, which means that it will travel all the way down to the colon.
2 The fiber does not travel alone; it carries along all the antioxidants, vitamins, and minerals found in the vegetables down to the colon, where they are used by the good bacteria.

Enzymes in the stomach and the small intestine simply haven't got the strength to digest most vegetable fiber, and therefore they let it pass untouched down to our Lukes, who receive them with gratitude. Once in the colon, the fiber is broken down by the good bacteria, which extract the nutrients and in turn provide them to our bodies.

As we mentioned earlier, the good bacteria can make use of the fiber to multiply and produce useful substances that help seal the intestines and protect against the leakage of toxins into the body, which strengthens our immune system further and protects us against different ailments.

Fig #5

IMPORTANT SOURCES OF WHOLESOME FIBER

(Source: Stig Bengmark)

Flaxseeds	Kiwi
Sunflower seeds	Raspberries
Passion fruit	Beets
Soy flour	Red cabbage
Avocado	White cabbage
Prunes	Gooseberries
Peanuts	Banana
Potatoes	Carrots
Hazelnuts (filberts)	Fennel
Blackberries	Savoy cabbage
Green peas	Blueberries
Pumpkin seeds	Cauliflower
Walnuts	Sprouts (i.e., bean sprouts)
Artichokes	Pears
Black currants	Strawberries
Onion	Tomatoes
Beans	Grapefruit
Brussels sprouts	Oranges
Olives	Apple (peel included)

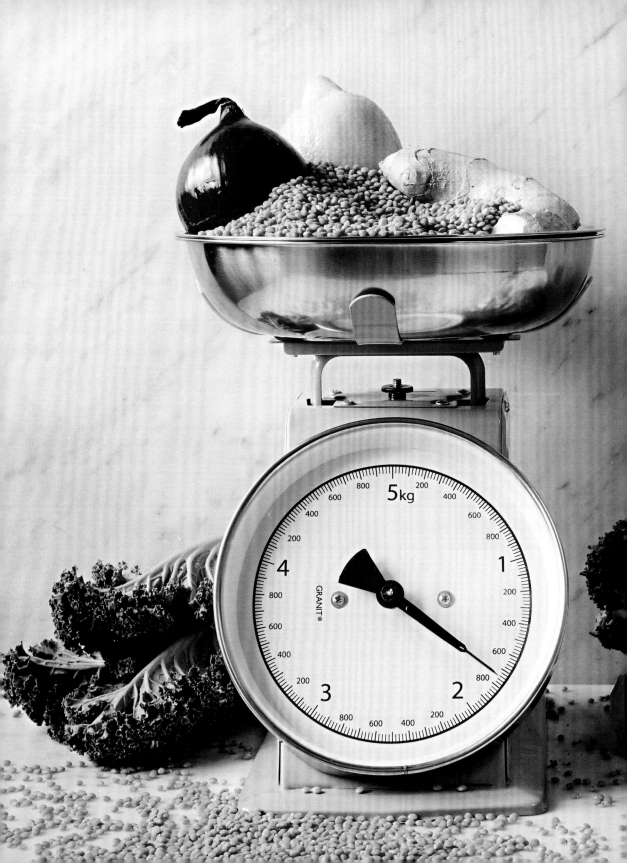

FOOD PHARMACY'S ALL-INCLUSIVE SOUP

(makes 2 large servings)

⅘ cup (200 ml) red lentils

1 tbsp vegetable stock powder

1 red onion, peeled

2 garlic cloves, peeled

3 stalks and heads of broccoli

Some kale

⅓ inch (1 cm) nub fresh ginger

Juice from ½ lemon

Salt and freshly ground black pepper

Chopped parsley

We make this soup several times a week. We usually boast that it's all-inclusive because you can vary it in infinite ways. You can use cauliflower and spinach instead of broccoli and kale, or swap the red onion for tomatoes, or use red lentils instead of the green ones . . . well, you get the idea. Start with what you already have in your refrigerator, and you will soon see how your life will change for the better.

Start by rinsing the lentils thoroughly, and boil them with the vegetable stock, prepared according to the package. While the lentils are cooking, chop the vegetables coarsely. Pull the soup pot off the heat and let it cool down for a few minutes. Add in the raw vegetables and spices. Use an immersion blender to puree the vegetables to the consistency of your liking. Stir in the lemon juice and sprinkle some parsley over the top, if you feel like it. Soup's on! the body, which strengthens our immune system further and protects us against different ailments.

We could say that fiber and intestinal bacteria are best buddies. Fiber is the most critical nutrient for good bacteria as it's strongly anti-inflammatory; many scientists argue that a lack of fiber is one of the major reasons we age prematurely.

INCREASE YOUR INTAKE OF FIBER GRADUALLY

Most of us eat too few vegetables and, unfortunately, too little fiber. Not many of us meet the USDA's recommended daily intake for fiber, which is 25–35 g per day. This is unfortunate, because the lack of fiber leads to a decrease in good bacteria, leaving the nasty bacteria to grow and thrive. To make matters worse, over time you will become less able to digest fiber if you consume too little of it. Intestinal flora that is not supplied with enough fiber can quite simply lose its fiber-digesting bacteria. Our ancestors, who ate much more fiber than we do, had much richer bacterial flora, both in the total amount of bacteria and the types of strains of bacteria. Today, many humans, especially those who suffer from increased inflammation, have significantly poorer intestinal flora.

Many people don't feel well after eating fiber, even though it is vital to our intestinal flora. They become bloated, experience abdominal pain, and suffer from flatulence and noisy intestines. It turns into a Catch-22, because that gas is a necessary part of the process, forming as good bacteria breaks down the fiber. As a result, it's very important to increase your fiber intake slowly to avoid such stomach issues. Some of us also get bellyaches when the fiber binds with water, which is why it's imperative to increase your water intake along with your fiber or you could get your tummy into trouble.

Try increasing your fiber intake gradually as you increase your fluid intake. If you still suffer from discomfort, the cause might be *irritable bowel syndrome* (IBS), a medical condition that plagues 25–45 million Americans. Remember that even if you suffer from IBS, the issues are very specific to each person, and symptoms can also vary and change over time. Nevertheless, fiber is vital.

Vitamin B_{12} is found primarily in animal products such as milk, meat, and eggs, so it's important that vegans take supplemental B_{12}. Our good bacteria do produce B_{12}, too, but in such variable quantities that if you're a strict vegan, it's still a good idea to take extra vitamin B_{12}.

THERE ARE TWO TYPES OF FIBER—SOLUBLE AND INSOLUBLE

Let's not leave the topic of fiber behind just yet.

Fiber is divided into two groups—soluble and insoluble. Since many of us have blood sugar levels that continuously ride a roller coaster, it's good to know that soluble fiber helps stabilize things. In other words, if you eat a lot of soluble fiber, it will affect the entire meal and keep your blood sugar more in balance, even if you eat something that has a high GI. Even though fiber doesn't contain any calories, it still promotes a heightened feeling of satiety. When soluble fiber is mixed with water, it forms a gel around the food we eat, which helps bulk up the stool to ease elimination. This makes food's passage through the intestine smoother, and it also helps the stomach empty more slowly.

Good sources for soluble fiber
Oat bran, berries, fruit, vegetables, lentils, chickpeas, figs, sunflower seeds, beans, flaxseed, sesame seed, and alfalfa seed.

Good sources for soluble fiber

Dennis Burkitt, a missionary and a surgeon, was an early researcher into the effects of fiber. While he worked in Uganda in the 1950s, he observed that most of the population who lived in the bush didn't suffer from most of the common ailments of the time, whether intestinal in nature (inflammatory intestinal diseases, for example) or those affecting the rest of the body (cardiovascular disease and diabetes). Burkitt began to measure the size of the stool and the time it took for food to travel through the body. He discovered that the size of European stool was about 60 g (2.11 oz) per twenty-four-hour cycle, compared to 600 g (21.1 oz) per twenty-four-hour cycle in Uganda, and that the time in transport took about a hundred hours in Europe compared to twenty hours in the African bush. Burkitt understood that the raw and completely unprocessed vegetable matter that made up much of the African diet hastened the passage of food through the intestine and saw that all the toxins were eliminated faster from the body.

Now we've come to the topic of insoluble fiber. The biggest difference between us (I'm talking about us here, Lina and Mia) and insoluble fiber is that the latter is like a neat-freak that loves to mop and clean up after itself. While we stretch out on the couch and leave the dinner dishes in the sink, insoluble fiber brushes away all toxins and debris from the intestine immediately and with great enthusiasm, while feeding large amounts of nutrients to the good bacteria at the same time.

Good sources for insoluble fiber

Good sources for insoluble fiber:
Leafy greens, whole grain products, and shells from many nuts and seeds.

We could call the colon our body's sewer system. Every day, this sewer system fills up with new toxins, such as dust, undigested food, heavy metals, pesticides, millions of dead cells, and who knows what else, and it's thanks to insoluble fiber that all this waste is ferried out of the body. Seen through a microscope, insoluble fiber looks like small sponges, which is very telling since we know how they work in the colon. Insoluble fiber can haul toxins several times its own size out of the body.

But to succeed in ridding the body of toxins, we need a lot of insoluble fiber. And when we say a lot, well, we mean a lot. Picture a sponge and you'll know what we're saying—there's quite a big difference between a sponge made from 5 g (0.17 oz) of fiber, and one that is made of 50 g (1.76 oz). The smaller the sponge, the more challenging it is to remove all the debris that collects in the drain.

THE EVEREST EFFECT

To be honest, we were both brought up in an environment where the conversation didn't often come around to poo, so when Professor Stig suddenly looked at us one day and proceeded enthusiastically and floridly to tell us about the Kebenkaise effect and its advantages, we quickly pricked up our ears and frantically began to take notes.

Everest is the highest mountain in Sweden. You can achieve the Everest effect by eating a lot of fiber, and the so-named "Everest sausage" is proof that you have ingested enough fiber. Everest is when the highest point of the stool in the toilet bowl breaks the water's surface, like the proud apex of an Alpine mountaintop. If the stool is too watery = no proud top. Also, if the stool is too hard = no proud top there, either. Poor fiber intake is directly reflected in the toilet bowl, and so if you wish to produce high-topped stool in the future, a high daily intake of fruit and vegetables is necessary (especially raw vegetables or unripe fruit). Another pearl of wisdom is that you should have trouble flushing the toilet completely in one go.

Let's try an experiment just for fun: we'll test the weight of our all-inclusive soup. We start out by setting a plate down on some scales, and spoon a mountain of red lentils on top. *What?* The scale displays only 200 g (7.05 oz). We continue by piling on some kale, garlic, and ginger, but the scale doesn't budge much even though we've added a big heap of vegetables. We add to this a boatload more of vegetables—half a head of broccoli, some red onion, and lemon, and a short while later we're over the finishing line, right at 700 g (about 3 to 4 cups).

Quinoa is some of the most antioxidant-rich food you can eat. Black quinoa is the most nutritious, followed by red and then white types.

Conclusions to be drawn from this experiment:
1 We eat far fewer vegetables than we originally thought.
2 We need to eat almost twice as many vegetables before the day is over.
3 We have to make a Everest-producing smoothie.

How do we do that? Get your blender out and we'll meet up again on the next page.

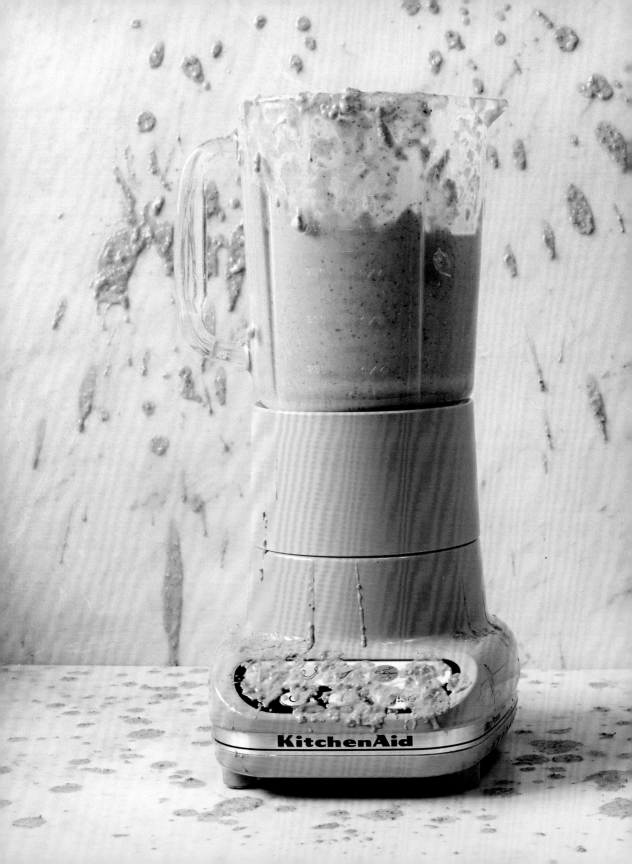

EVEREST SMOOTHIE

(makes 2 glasses)

2½ oz (70 g) leafy greens
(arugula or mâche, for example)

2 handfuls baby spinach

½ hothouse (English) cucumber

½ lemon, peeled

¾ inch (2 cm) nub fresh ginger

2 stalks celery

1 avocado

⁴/₅ cup (200 ml) water

1 tbsp coconut oil

This smoothie is full of yummy vegetable fiber that goes all the way down to your protective bacteria in the colon. In addition, this smoothie is alkaline, thanks to the leafy greens, cucumber, and lemon. Its flavor is green and fresh, and if this smoothie doesn't make you (and us) produce Everest-style tops like a conveyer belt, we'll be very disappointed.

Put everything in the blender and press the start button. Stop when you have a soft smoothie in the pitcher. Here's to tops!

Instead of juicing it, add the lemon peel to the smoothie. That way, you reap all benefits from the vegetables' fiber and enjoy an extra-large dose of antioxidants from the lemon's white pith.

FOCUS ON LEAFY GREENS

The USDA's recommendation that we eat at least 2½–3 cups of vegetables per day can, of course, be interpreted in several ways. If you're a bit of a nerd and like to take things literally, you could take 2½ cups of beets and shove them into your mouth. Unfortunately, it isn't quite so simple.

Because all plant food has been thrown together under one umbrella term—*vegetables*—it becomes rather misleading to illustrate how much one needs to eat by using a volume or weight measure. From a purely nutritional standpoint, it might be more correct to concentrate a bit less on unit measurement, and instead choose vegetables based on their highest possible nutritional density. Take leafy greens, for example. No matter how much kale, chard, and spinach you pile on your plate, they still don't weigh very much, but they're far more nutrient-dense than those beets.

There's no quibble that leafy greens are among the best foods you can eat. First, they're rich in vitamins and minerals, and they're chock-full of magnesium, which our protective bacteria need in order to multiply. Second, green leaves contain a huge amount of insoluble fiber (you know, the sponges). Third, they contain the unusual sugar molecule SQ (Sulfoquinovese) which prevents bad bacteria from colonizing the colon and helps the good bacteria thrive. Finally, the green color broadcasts that the leaves are full of chlorophyll, which provides good bacteria with oxygen and in turn allows the bacteria to grow and increase in number (it also seems that bad bacteria can't tolerate oxygen in gas form). We're having a hard time holding ourselves back, but here's just one more advantage, a fifth: they are so *alkaline*. Today, it's more the rule than the exception that we humans skew toward acidic levels, and an acidic environment is the ideal condition for bad bacteria to multiply.

SCIENCE FOR YOU

Don't forget to eat different varieties of leafy greens, since the amounts of different nutrients vary across the different types of greens.

SPRUCE UP YOUR SPICE CABINET

Spices are loaded with antioxidants, and they're an extremely effective shield against inflammation. Antioxidants are, as you may

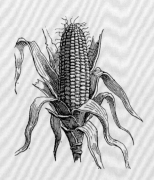

HOW WELL DOES YOUR COLON WORK? HERE ARE THREE SIMPLE TESTS YOU CAN PERFORM TO FIND OUT.

01. The Jerusalem artichoke test. The Jerusalem artichoke is very rich in wholesome but hard-to-digest fiber called fructans. If you can eat an entire raw, average-sized Jerusalem artichoke without experiencing any discomfort, your intestinal flora is not bad.

02. The Everest test. If your intestinal flora is working well, it's normal to have stools weighing just under one pound (about 400 to 500 g) twice daily. However, modern toilets are not built for this, so count on your toilet becoming slightly overworked. A small "Alpine tip" should peak over the water line, and the water should rise a little when you flush the toilet.

03. The corn test. In a perfect world, waste's journey through the body should take about twenty-four hours (up to forty-eight hours is okay). You can check this by keeping an eye out for when the corn kernels reappear.

SCIENCE FOR YOU

We separate seasonings into herbs and spices. Herbs come from the vegetables' leaves, while spices or seasonings come from other parts of the plants, such as the roots, stem, seeds, pips, fruits, or berries.

AND

Make treats wholesome by seasoning berries, nuts, and fruit with cinnamon, cardamom, cloves, ginger, and cocoa. Not only do they taste heavenly, they're also some of the most antioxidant-rich spices in existence.

recall, the body's primary defense against free radicals, and as such they protect the body against inflammation, illness, and aging. Antioxidants are also important components in epigenetics and can protect you by preventing an inherited gene from becoming active. When vegetable fiber reaches the colon, your small Lukes extract antioxidants from the vegetables and make sure that they get out into the body.

Scientists commonly measure the effect of antioxidants using *ORAC* (Oxygen Radical Absorbation Capacity), a measure that quantifies the concentration of antioxidants and their ability to deal with free radicals. Spices often contain more antioxidants per gram than other parts of the plant. While it is primarily different types of spices that make it to the top of ORAC's list, you'll also find sorghum, acai berries, quinoa, and sumac in the top tier of antioxidant-rich foods.

We filled our entire kitchen with spices as soon as we realized that many of them were on ORAC's best-of list. Dried spices went into the spice cabinet and fresh herbs went into pots, as well as in the refrigerator and freezer. Antioxidant levels were boosted in simple, everyday meals when we seasoned our dinners with cumin, parsley, turmeric, black pepper, oregano, dill, rosemary, and coriander. We also quickly noted which spices were a hit with the kids and used them liberally when we served a new dish we worried they might not want to try. Another discovery was that we didn't need to add as much salt as before, salt being our go-to seasoning for everything in the past.

Unfortunately, the formula isn't that simple—not every nutrient-dense food is automatically anti-inflammatory. Take beans for example, which we often eat and which are very nutritious: they're healthy for intestinal flora but also slightly inflammatory. We're not hardliners, but a good tip is to get into the habit of seasoning inflammatory foods with anti-inflammatory spices.

Fig, #6

FOOD IN ALL THE COLORS OF THE RAINBOW

Red
Tomatoes, red bell peppers, cherries, chili peppers, cranberries, raspberries, strawberries, radishes, red currants, pomegranate, rhubarb, ruby grapefruit, blood oranges, watermelon, lingonberries

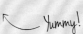
Yummy!

Yellow/orange
Oranges, yellow bell peppers, cloudberries, carrots, melon, pineapple, peaches, persimmons, ground cherries (physalis), pumpkin, mangoes, apricots, rutabaga (swede), grapefruit, lemons, papaya, passion fruit

Blue/lilac
Blueberries, blackberries, black currants, grapes, red cabbage, red onion, plums, eggplant, figs, beets

Green
Spinach, broccoli, kale, lettuce chard, avocado, Jerusalem artichokes, asparagus, Brussels sprouts, nettles, savoy cabbage, chili peppers, green bell peppers, peas, kiwi, leeks, limes, sugar snap peas, basil, zucchini, pears, apples, celery, grapes, fennel

White/brown
Parsnips, onions, garlic, potatoes, Jerusalem artichokes, bananas, dark chocolate containing more than 70 percent cocoa, dates, raisins, white cabbage, coconut, litchi, mangosteens, black radishes, parsley root, mushrooms, cauliflower

---

THINK OF IT AS A SMALL ANTIOXIDANT RAINBOW

We always carry a mental image of a rainbow with us when we shop for and prepare food. *A rainbow?* Yes, because you should always mix three colors together when you eat fruit and vegetables. This phenomenon is called rainbow foods. Antioxidants in the form of phytochemicals are in all fruit and vegetable colors; they act as the plants' immune system and are critical to their survival because they protect them from UV radiation and against attacks from viruses, bacteria, and different kinds of pollution. They exhibit powerful antioxidant characteristics.

Different colors contain different types of phytochemicals and they all have varying positive effects on our health. So, if you eat only green vegetables, you'll only reap the benefit from the phytochemicals found in green veggies. Many phytochemicals only protect against specific free radicals, so to gain the most out of them it's important to eat a good mix of different types of vegetables, fruit, berries, and nuts, and not just live day in and day out on carrots and cashews. If you eat from a wider color palette—orange, red, and green, for instance—you'll take in a variety of phytochemicals that strengthen each other, too.

An interesting fact is that 1 + 1 doesn't necessarily add up to 2 in the world of phytochemicals. Since different phytochemicals reinforce each other's properties, this sometimes means that 1 + 1 = 3. That's why it's a good rule of thumb to always feature several colors of the vegetable kingdom in your meal; this will provide your body with a secure, wall-to-wall carpet of disease-inhibitors. Just remember to think "rainbow" next time you're standing there, indecisive, in front of the refrigerator, and everything will be just fine.

Berries, apples, green bananas, peaches, and apricots are good fruits to add to a green smoothie to help neutralize an overly strong flavor.

EAT WHAT OTHERS THROW AWAY

Traditionally, humans have always eaten the least nutritious part of a plant. Nutrients in fruit and vegetables are not as equally distributed throughout as we would imagine. When we choose carrots for dinner, it's a real shame that we discard the nutrient-rich green tops instead of chowing down on them, too.

Do you recall from the last chapter that humans have typically only eaten flour, which is the least nutrient-dense part of the grain? The same applies to the green tops of all root vegetables, which usually end up in the garbage, even though those green tops are less calorific, have low fat or sugar content, and have much more vital fiber and many more minerals and vitamins than the root vegetable itself. This is also true for the fruits we enjoy each day: the most nutritious parts of the apple and pear are those we habitually don't eat: the pips, the core, and the peel.

Speaking of wasting food, we often use the freezer to both reduce waste and preserve nutrients. Research on lettuce has shown that its ORAC value is cut in half by as quickly as half an hour after the leaves were separated from the root. It is therefore an advantage to freeze the green tops of vegetables if you don't plan on eating them that day—in doing so, you'll preserve their nutrients and their antioxidant qualities (their ORAC content).

A SMOOTHIE IS ALWAYS HEALTHIER THAN JUICE

One of the most important yet simple changes we've made since we set off on this pilgrim's journey is to drink one green smoothie a day. This way, we get to gorge on leafy greens and easily reap all the benefits from the vegetables' most nutritious parts. Smoothies are the solution to everything (except marital strife, political crises, and financial burdens). Sometimes a smoothie will replace lunch, some days we drink it as an energizer, and now and then we do as Professor Stig does and have one instead of dinner. You know, for those days when you can't muster the energy to fix a meal and would typically reach for the bread and butter instead. Those days.

A blender is the perfect tool if you want to keep all the nutrients in vegetables (mostly in green leaves). The nutrients are stored in the cells of leaves, and to extract them you need to either 1) chew very thoroughly and at length (which most of us usually never take the time to do), or 2) use a blender, which breaks down the cellulose to release the nutrients.

Don't forget to add the pips and the green tops to your smoothie. However, one exception is rhubarb leaves! They're toxic!

More advantages to smoothies:
You can eat lots of vegetables and leafy greens without a fight.

1 You don't need to chop anything (good if you're in a hurry or if your arm is in a sling).
2 You don't have to chew (good if you're in a hurry or if you have braces on your teeth).
3 You don't need to do any dishes (especially if you drink straight out of the pitcher).
4 You can, in fact, lie on the couch and imbibe it (you might need a straw for that, though).

However, do not confuse smoothies with juice. Fresh-pressed juice is currently hotter than it's ever been, but, really, its newfound hipness is undeserved. There are three things that indicate that juice doesn't live up to all the health hype it has garnered, and those are its sugar content, lack of vitamins, and lack of fiber.

The difference between green juice and a green smoothie is that the smoothie contains the entire vegetable, whereas the juice consists of only the juice from the vegetable. The reason juiced vegetables and fruits are worse for the body than a smoothie is quite simply because with juicing, the fiber (peel, core, and fruit flesh) disappears, which makes its sugar unhealthier. Smoothies and juice yield the same amount of sugar but affect health, blood sugar, intestinal flora, and inflammation in different ways. Just like the case of warm potatoes from the last chapter!

If we attempted to establish an order of priority on how to eat raw fruits and vegetables, these would be the guidelines:

1 Preferably, eat vegetables and fruit in their natural state.
2 Opt for smoothies instead of juices (that way, you get the vital fiber). This is a great way to get a whole lot of vegetables!
3 In the ideal world, pick vegetable juice, which contains less sugar, over fruit juice; and skip store-bought "fresh-pressed" juice.
4 At this point, we're wracking our brains but we can't find another health-related argument. Basically, skip all juices and don't give them to your children—that is, if you're giving juice to them because of their so-called health benefits.

SCIENCE FOR YOU

A random sample of grapes from the European Union contained twenty-six different types of pesticides. It might be a good idea to opt for something else if you can't find organic grapes, raisins, or wine.

DEVOTE THE LARGEST SECTION OF YOUR PLATE TO VEGETABLES

Ahem, do you think we're trying to convert you to veganism now? Nah, not quite . . . well, maybe?

For environmental reasons, a lot of people should decrease their intake of meat. We are taking a more serious tone here (cue the violin strings): worldwide meat consumption has tripled over the past forty years. Even countries like India and China (where most of the planet's population live), where people traditionally ate very little meat, are starting to copy our First World meat- and dairy-centric dietary habits. Additionally, the meat industry has become the villain behind one of humanity's most current and biggest health crises: multidrug-resistant bacteria. Most antibiotics in use today are not prescribed for humans but given to animals reared for meat production (Sweden is the exception to this rule). Keep in mind that meat consumption alone is one of the largest contributors of greenhouse gases, which in turn is one of the biggest threats to our existence here on Earth.

From the short-term view of intestinal flora: no, you don't have to become a vegan. But if most of us don't decrease our intake of meat, our world will not survive, and our intestinal flora will go down along with it.

Lina looks unhappily out of a train window. Mia casually flips through a magazine.

– Hey, this a funny article. Look!

– I can't read when I'm on the train, it makes me sick as a dog.

– Okay. Anyway, it's a weird article about what our Christmas dinner table will look like in 2050. They're saying that Christmas ham will be made from beans and algae, and casseroles will consist of protein-rich insects and larvae.

Lina continues to concentrate on the pine trees.

– Ha ha! It says here that we will feast on real, old-fashioned beef loin with Béarnaise sauce on Christmas Day. "It's going to cost a fortune because animal protein will be climate-taxed through the roof—but for dinner out once a year, it'll be worth it."

Still concentrating . . .

– Our grandchildren will probably find it truly strange that only a few years ago humans got access to plant nutrients by way of animal stomachs. What do you think?

We make a point of not eating corn on the cob. Corn is one of the most over-processed—and now GMO-manipulated—foods on Earth. Furthermore, corn contains the protein zein, which blocks the storage of the necessary amino acid tryptophan, which is needed to make the neurotransmitter serotonin (which in turn affects worry, anxiety, satiation, and pain) and melatonin (which affects biorhythm, alertness, and sleep).

Lina takes her eyes off the pines and looks at Lina.
– Mia, I don't believe anything right now. Actually, I believe I'm going to puke.
Lina gets up and rushes to the toilet.

LET'S CLEAR UP THREE MYTHS ABOUT MEAT AND DAIRY PRODUCTS

We go all out when it comes to choosing organic food. Keep in mind that organic meat can come from animals that have been fed conventionally-raised grains and concentrates.

Myth 1: You will not get enough protein. Let's take it from the top. Protein used to be called the "building blocks" of the body because it is used to repair and build new body cells and tissue. Protein is made up of eight essential amino acids (nine in children), which need to be acquired through diet. Animal protein contains all the essential amino acids and is therefore called a complete protein, compared to the protein found in plants, which do not have all essential amino acids. This doesn't mean you can't get complete protein because you're a vegan; you just need to be more mindful to combine different sources of vegetarian protein and eat larger amounts of it (because the body has an easier time using up animal protein than vegetable protein). You don't have to worry about not getting enough protein if you eat a large salad that includes lots of leafy greens, nuts, buckwheat, and legumes.

Examples of vegetarian protein sources:
Grains, legumes, leafy greens, sorghum, brewer's yeast, seeds, and buckwheat.

Mia stares through the window of a train.
– Next stop: Gothenburg.
Lina puts on her jacket. Mia doesn't move a muscle.
– In any case, it's interesting because I always believed that only animal protein was effective . . . especially when it comes to building muscle.
– Hmmm . . .
– Where do you think bulls get their muscles from?
– Huh?

– Do you think it's because they've drunk a lot of protein-enriched milk?
– I really don't know, Lina, I'm not feeling that great . . .
– Or because they've loaded up on grilled salmon?
– Can you please stop talking about food . . .
The train pulls into the terminal. Mia stands up and rushes to the toilet.

Myth 2: You will not get enough iron.
Iron deficiency affects more than one quarter of the world's population
(and it can affect you, whether you're vegan or not). It's true that vegans
and vegetarians tend to suffer from iron deficiency in larger numbers than
omnivores, but if you're aware of this it's easy to fulfill your requirement for
iron even with a vegan diet.

It's fortunate that many protein-rich vegetables are also rich in iron. Iron
is a bit difficult for the body to absorb, but many vegetables and fruits contain
vitamin C, which facilitates bioavailability. If you include fermented foods
in your meal, your body will have an easier time taking in iron and other
minerals.

Examples of iron-rich food:
Broccoli, beans, chia seeds, wheat germ, sesame seeds, nuts, spinach, nettles,
and chickpeas.

Myth 3: You will not get enough calcium.
Uh—hello? Did you grow up in a country where milk is sacrosanct? Milk lobbies
in many Western countries like America and Sweden, where we grew up, are
very strong, and that's why studies listing the health-giving properties of milk
are given more airtime than those suggesting that a high intake of milk might
not be all that great for us. It's been drilled into us since childhood that milk
gives us strong bones, but in all honesty it's been a long time since milk was
the best source of calcium available to us. Even though Americans and Swedes
are one of the greatest consumers of milk in the world, they also suffer some of
the highest rates of bone fractures in the world. Recent scientific research even
links higher risk of fractures to drinking milk.

Last year, the Swedish Food Agency lowered the recommended intake of
milk because many studies now show that large quantities of milk contribute
to ill health. As for our intestinal flora, it doesn't exactly crave milk, either.

On the contrary, consuming large quantities of dairy-rich products and saturated fat contributes to an increase of inflammation in the body.

Examples of calcium-rich food:
Kale, parsley, rosehip, sesame seeds, almonds, brown beans/bush beans, white beans, arugula, spinach, Brazil nuts, nettles, and garlic.

Go ahead and buy frozen spices and herbs. It's very economical, and they're just as nutritious as their fresh counterparts.

THERE IS A CORRELATION BETWEEN MEAT AND INFLAMMATION

By the end of 2015, the WHO (World Health Organization) changed its recommendations and reclassified red meat—processed meats in particular—as carcinogenic to humans. This was the first time the WHO had called a food cancer-causing, and since many of us eat red meat and processed meat daily, articles were published everywhere and it became widespread news. This meant that bacon, sausage, and ready-to-eat meatballs are now on the same list of shame as asbestos and tobacco. That list is called "Group 1: Carcinogenic to humans," which implies that the scientific evidence against these products is the same (however, it's important to point out that this does not mean that the risk for cancer is identical for each product within Group 1).

 – *Woof! What does that mean?*
 Lina's dog Pyret is startled awake and looks up confusedly from her basket. Maybe it's just my imagination, but it looks like she can't quite figure out how this could work, because she still sees Lina and Mia serving meat from time to time. Lina looks to Mia for help, and Mia takes the lead.
 – *Well, you see, Pyret, it's like this . . .*

As you've probably figured out by now, we eat a primarily plant-based diet, but we haven't given up meat altogether. From our intestinal flora's perspective, as well as from Professor Stig's, it's perfectly fine to eat up to 33 lb (15 kg) of meat per year (about 10.5 oz or 300 g per week). The USDA's Dietary Guidelines recommends that we eat 25–35 oz of meat per week, but this recommendation has faced criticism for not limiting meat intake enough. The Swedish National Food Agency advises that we eat no more than 16 oz of meat per week, and Britain's Food Standards Agency draws the line lower at no more than 10.5 oz per week. Scientific proof that your general health will be improved by abstaining from eating meat entirely just isn't in yet. There are many things to take into consideration—what the animals are being fed, how the meat is cooked, how much of it we consume, etc.—but it seems that enjoying meat in limited quantities is not harmful. In large quantities, however, meat will give Darth and his army plenty of ammunition.

In the ideal world, the following applies:
1 Occasionally abstain from eating meat, or cut down on the frequency with which you serve it.
2 When you do eat meat, make sure to choose organic and grass-fed, pasture-raised meat. (Sadly, even some types of game are fed conventional supplemental feed these days.)
3 Do not eat processed meat. It's important that the meat you buy be organic and clean, i.e., not processed or prepared ahead.

And in the real world? By all means, challenge yourself a little. Try to make vegetables the stars on your plate a few times a week. Prepare vegetarian versions of your most frequent meals (if you use the same seasoning, it usually works fine). Make a lot of soup. Swap the ham and the liver paté on a sandwich with nut butter and avocado. And if you want your children to eat more vegetables, don't tell them to do it, but lead by example.

After all this, it's time to prepare our favorite dip.

Turn the page and we'll take it from there.

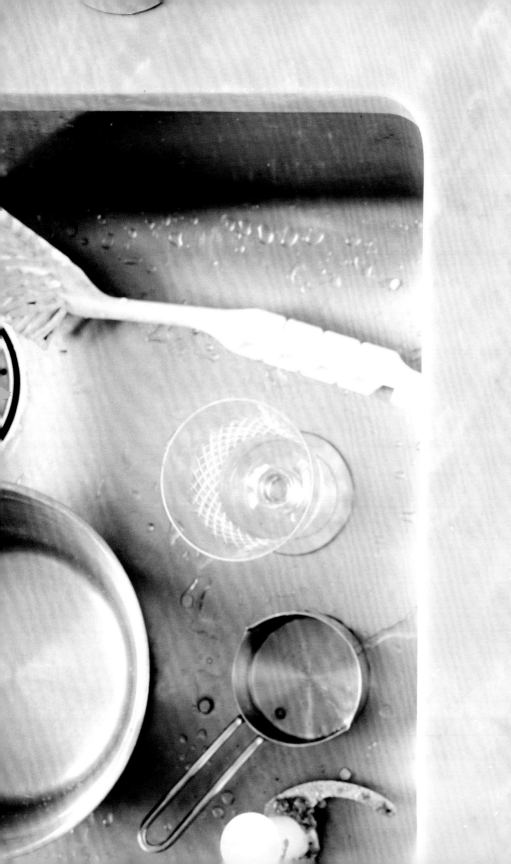

CARROT TOP PASTA PESTO

(makes 2 servings)

ANTI-INFLAMMATORY • FOR YOU •

3 large carrots

²/₅ cup (100 ml) carrot tops

1 garlic clove

²/₅ cup (100 ml) basil leaves

²/₅ cup (100 ml) hazelnuts (filberts)

1 tbsp freshly squeezed lemon juice

¹/₅ cup (50 ml) olive oil

Salt and freshly ground black pepper

This pesto is extra healthy due to the inclusion of some unusual vegetable parts. As in, using the carrot tops instead of the root. It's so nutrient-dense that half a serving is enough. Say what? What should we do with the carrot? Turn it into spaghetti, of course!

Pull off the carrot tops and chop them coarsely. Mix them with garlic, basil leaves, hazelnuts, and lemon juice. Add olive oil in a thin stream until the pesto thickens. Season with salt and pepper. Use a potato peeler, mandolin, or vegetable spiralizer to make long spaghetti-like strands with the carrot onto an attractive plate. Top with the pesto!

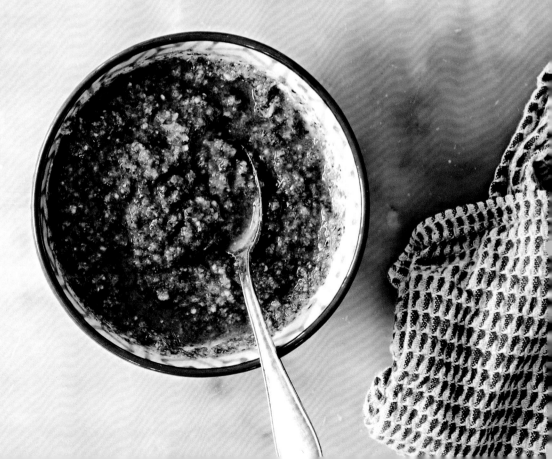

Food Pharmacy's Favorite #6

KALE

Unfortunately, there hasn't been as much research on cabbage as there should be, but to be diplomatic, kale is strongly believed to alleviate inflammation, strengthen the immune system, and boost metabolism, since it contains everything from iron, omega-3, fiber, and vitamins A, C, and K to minerals and antioxidants.

We can also tell you that kale is an excellent source of calcium. So, next time we want some calcium, we'll skip the milk and toss a few handfuls of kale in the soup instead.

(However, we won't do this to coffee. We must set boundaries somewhere.)

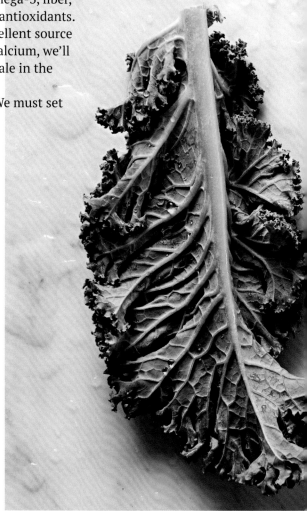

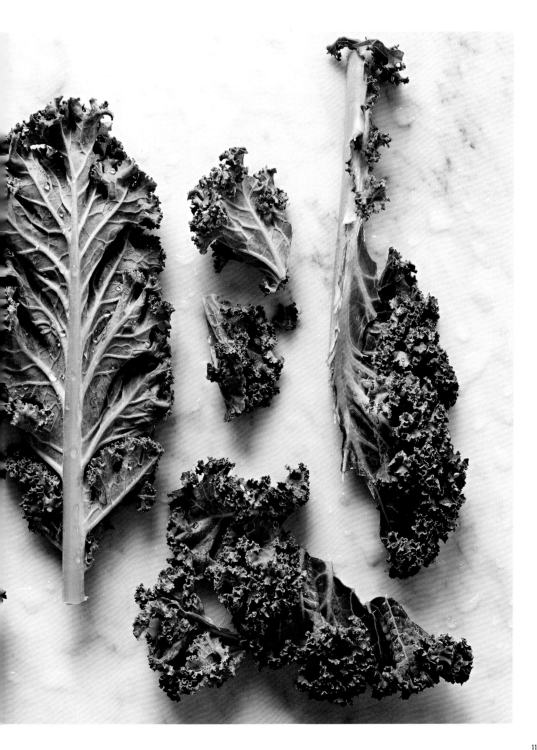

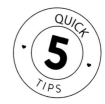

A brief summary about gorging on vegetables:

FIVE GREEN TIPS FOR INTESTINAL FLORA

01. Start by checking out the produce aisle. Try a new vegetable the next time you shop.

02. Make one of our green smoothies. If it tastes too green for your taste, just add an apple.

03. Find out what you like. You don't like raw broccoli? Try steaming it. Or season it with sea salt and olive oil.

04. Make a salad and top it with different goodies such as seeds, nuts, olive oil, and lemon.

05. Add yummy dips to your meal! Mix up some hummus with chickpeas, garlic, olive oil, and parsley, or some guacamole with avocado, garlic, tomato, lime, and heaps of fresh cilantro.

CHOOSE YOUR FATS WISELY

(and give the inflammation a run for its money)

We've come to our book's first fish recipe. Fact: fatty fish is known to inhibit inflammation. Mackerel is a great source of the essential fatty acid omega-3, and research has shown that fish oils provide strong protection against all chronic illnesses that inflammation has a hand in.

In general, fish—and fatty fish specifically—contain lots of fatty acids called DHA (Doxosahexaenoic acid) and EPA (Eicosapentaenoic acid) that are easily absorbed by the body. Recent animal research has shown that if we're scrupulous about getting our omega-3s, we'll have considerably better intestinal flora and reduce levels of inflammation-causing and poisonous endotoxin in the body. Let's hear it—more mackerel for the people.

OUR FAT CV (CURRICULUM VITAE)

A few decades ago, the alarm was sounded: fat makes us sick and overweight. Scientists all over the world connected obesity with saturated fat, and one morning when we came down to breakfast, the red carton of milk was suddenly yellow, and the container of butter had flowers on it.

Us, as kids: "Morning. What's with the milk carton and the butter?"
Our moms: "Ah, come and sit down. Try this new fat-free milk and the light margarine."

We happily began to experiment with different low-fat dieting methods—not because we needed to lose weight, necessarily, but because, well, everyone was doing it, right? For us, the 1980s and 90s were very much about how to eat to control our weight, and not at all about how food made us feel. If you could button the top of your Levi's 501, you were free to eat as much ice cream and cinnamon buns as you wanted. But if you couldn't fasten that button, it was time to get on that fat-free diet. And the diet that was the lowest in fat had to be the Flight Attendant's Diet.

The Flight Attendant's Diet was the diet to end all diets, and it had you cutting out fat completely. Naturally, it wasn't only fat that we cut out; it was almost everything. Breakfast would consist of half a grapefruit. Advantage: you could lose eleven pounds and fit into your jeans for a little while. Drawback: You were ravenously hungry, suffered from horrific headaches, and gained all the weight back (and then some) as soon as you started eating normally again.

WE EAT TOO MUCH OF THE WRONG KINDS OF FAT

Today, we know it wasn't fat that caused our weight problem, and it's such a shame that our fear of fat had the opportunity to wreak such havoc. Between 1990 and 2000, the number of obese people in the Western world increased from two to three hundred million, and many think this trend correlates directly to changes people made when they began to avoid saturated fat. People started consuming oils rich in polyunsaturated omega-6 fatty acids, as well as processed food full of hydrogenated fats and trans fats. Nobody knew at the time that they were increasing their risk of free radicals and inflammation in the body. We're aware of this now, and yet these fats still comprise more than half of our intake of fat, at just over 88 lb (40 kg) per person per year.

All our organs require fat, especially our brain and cardiovascular system. Fat is necessary for our body to absorb fat-soluble vitamins (A, D, E, and K), and don't forget that fat lowers our meals' glycemic index, too. At least 20–30 percent of the food you eat should be some type of fat.

Before we got to know Professor Stig, we thought we had our fat consumption down pat; we knew it wasn't bad for us. But then, as usual, whenever we visited Stig in Höganäs, we learned something new. Stig confirmed that fat is indeed vital, but this does not grant us license to overdose on the stuff. "Everything in moderation," as he likes to say. He also taught us that there's a difference between fats: some fats are bad for intestinal flora, and other fats are good for it; and our problem is that we consume too little of the healthy fat and way too much of the wrong fats. The latter category primarily includes all the animal fats and omega-6s that, when consumed in large quantities, are strongly linked to inflammation.

Fats are typically divided into the following groups:

1 Saturated fat (found in butter, full-fat dairy products, processed meats, coconut oil)
2 Monounsaturated fat (found in olive oil, flaxseed oil, and walnuts)
3 Hydrogenated fat, which is simply polyunsaturated fat that has been turned into saturated fat through the process of industrial food production (found in French fries, cookies, instant gravy and sauces, candy, and microwaveable popcorn)

Many different fats can coexist in one single product. Butter, for example, is considered a saturated fat, but it contains some unsaturated fat as well. Fat can also be made up of short-, medium-, or long-chained fatty acids. Butter counts as a long-chain acid fat, but it has a small amount of short- and medium-chain fatty acids, too. To complicate things further, two saturated fats can have fatty acids of different lengths. For example, butter and coconut oil are two saturated fats, but butter has long-chain fatty acids and coconut oil has medium-chain fatty acids. To simplify, we can say that short-chain fatty acids put less stress on the body than their long-chained counterparts.

Two polyunsaturated fatty acids are essential fatty acids. They are commonly classified as omega-3 and omega-6.

THE VITAL OMEGA-3 AND OMEGA-6 FATS

There are also *essential fatty acids,* which are, as their name implies, indispensable. Unfortunately, the body is unable to manufacture these by itself, so we need to procure them from outside sources via our diet. Alpha-linolenic acid (mom to omega-3s) and linolenic acid (mom to omega-6s) are both crucial and are important for, among other things, building cell walls and controlling inflammation in the body. Omega-3s are always healthy: they inhibit inflammation, while omega-6s can be two-faced, since they can either inhibit and abet inflammation. If too much omega-6 is ingested along with too little omega-3, the omega-6s will turn into an inflammatory fatty acid.

At the same time, omega-6s are vital and healthy if ingested in appropriate amounts.

Omega-3s can come from either two sources: the ocean (DHA and EPA) or plants (ALA). There are large amounts of DHA and EPA in fatty fish such as mackerel, herring, and salmon. In plants, we find omega-3s primarily in leafy greens (an excellent excuse to drink a daily green smoothie), flaxseeds, and walnuts. In nature, omega-6s are found primarily in seeds and nuts.

The best plant sources for omega-3s:
Leafy greens, walnuts, chia seeds, rapeseed oil, and whole flaxseeds (preferably freshly crushed with a pestle and mortar right before eating, but limit to 1–2 tablespoons per day).

OBS

As mentioned before, to keep inflammation in check it's important to keep an eye on the balance of omega-3s to omega-6s. In our ancestors' diet, the ratio was often 1:1, and many scientists believe that since our genetic makeup is slow to evolve, our bodies are probably at their best if we apply that same proportion today. A small amount of these fatty acids is plenty, so long as their balance is right. Today, however, we're ingesting tiny quantities of omega-3s and large amounts of omega-6s, a state of affairs that saddens Luke and makes Darth happy; that weakens the immune system and stimulates chronic inflammation and chronic diseases. On the next page, we'll share with you some of our favorite recipes for boosting the body's immune system using omega-3s from the sea.

WHY IS THE BALANCE OF OMEGA-3 AND OMEGA-6 UNEVEN?

Following the lead of scientists, who for so many years warned us against saturated fat, the food industry began mass-producing different types of polyunsaturated oils. As omega-3s are a very delicate fatty acid that can easily turn rancid, it was more profitable to ignore omega-3 fats and

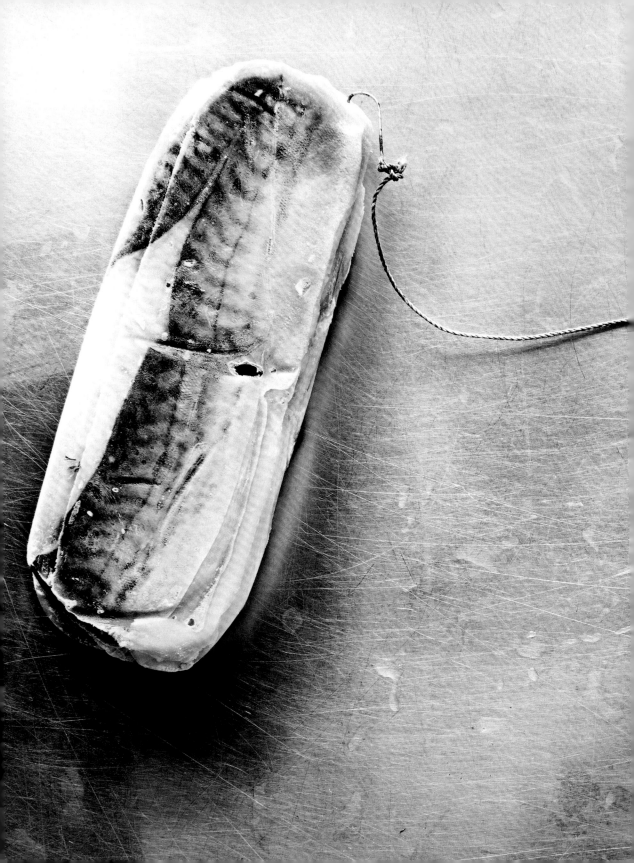

ANTI-INFLAMMATORY OVEN-BAKED MACKEREL WITH HERBS AND RAW LINGONBERRY JAM

(serves 4)

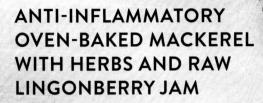

Mackerel	Raw lingonberry jam
¾ lb (400 g) frozen mackerel	1³/₅ cup (400 ml) lingonberries
Dill, fresh or frozen	4 dates
Black pepper	

Mackerel is a big favorite in our house. During wintertime, we have no option but to fish it out of the freezer, but in the summer, which we spend on the Swedish west coast, we enjoy freshly caught fish. We pile into the boat with Grandpa, a few kids, a thermos of coffee, and patience. Sometimes the fish bite, sometimes not. But who cares about that when you're on vacation and you spent the day on the beach?

Defrost the mackerel. Preheat the oven to 160°F (71°C). Place the fillets in an ovenproof dish and sprinkle with dill and pepper. Slide the fish in the oven and wait until the fish has reached 130°F (54°C). If you don't have an oven thermometer at your disposal, you'll have to trust your own judgment—it usually takes around half an hour or thereabouts. Mix the lingonberries and dates. Serve the mackerel with lingonberries and cooled potatoes.

increase food's shelf-life by manufacturing cheaper oils rich in the hardier omega-6 fatty acids instead. These oils aren't merely taking up shelf space with the rest of the oils at the grocery store; they're also in just about every industrially manufactured food product available. That's how the healthy ratio between vital fatty acids has been upset, and why we ingest far too much omega-6 and far too little omega-3.

Omega-3 becomes rancid very quickly, which makes these fatty acids go from healthy to harmful. Store walnuts, flaxseeds, and other omega-3 rich nuts and seeds in a dark and cool environment, like in your refrigerator. Also, store oils in a dark and cool place and make sure that the lid is on tight.

Lina and Mia are at McDonald's. Just kidding. Lina and Mia are visiting the Royal Library in Stockholm, and are each enjoying a glass of water.

– Mia, have you ever heard of ILSI?

– No, what's that?

– It's a global research network. The letters stand for the International Life Science Institute, which is overseen by the food industry and multinational corporations such as Coca-Cola and Nestlé. And now they're in the British Journal of Nutrition and are saying that . . .

Lina makes small "rabbit ear" air quotes with her fingers.

– . . . without a doubt, low-grade inflammation is connected to a long line of lifestyle diseases in the Western world.

Mia looks up from her New York Times *and pushes her glasses down her nose.*

– Well, that's exciting!

Lina closes her issue of the British Journal of Nutrition.

– And in the next sentence they go on to say that there's a correlation between low-grade inflammation and bad fats and carbohydrates. So let's hope they'll invest in making better products that will make us healthy instead of sick.

– Sure . . . but in the meantime, I'll keep buying clean and unprocessed food. If we keep that as our mantra while perusing the aisles, we don't need to worry about added sugars, processed carbohydrates, inflammatory fats, or foods with antibiotics and pesticide residue.

Our future Nobel prize–winners lean back in their chairs and sigh contentedly.

In hindsight, it's easy to feel kind of sad at the thought of so many people switching from saturated fat to vegetable oils with high levels of omega-6s. Because omega-6s slow down people's metabolisms, many ended up putting on weight instead of losing it when they made the switch. However, the main fallout from the increased consumption of omega-6s is that the crucial balance between omega-3s and omega-6s was upended.

Furthermore, polyunsaturated oils are extremely delicate and have low smoke points, which leads to the formation of carcinogenic substances when those oils are heated up. When we began to fry our foods in oil instead of butter, we suddenly ingested more carcinogenic matter.

This balance is also disrupted in our fish and meat supplies. Historically, we used to ingest a good mix of omega-3s and omega-6s because the animals we ate got their fatty acids from their respective natural sources: grass and plankton. Unfortunately, now most of the animals we consume are bred for the food industry and are fed concentrated feed and grains instead of straw and grass, so their meat contains an excess of omega-6s. Meat from grass-fed animals and game is still rich in omega-3s, and this also applies to farmed fish that is not fed with grain. The source of omega-3s in fish comes from the chlorophyll that small fish get by eating phytoplankton, and wild-caught fish is rich in omega-3s. But as soon as the fish are fed grains, they will have unnatural amounts of omega-6s instead of their naturally large quantities of omega-3s.

Only part of the ALA (omega-3s from plants) can be transformed into DNA and EPA, which we find in fatty fish. For that reason, you should take an omega-3 supplement (containing DNA and EPA) if you don't eat fish.

CHOOSE THE RIGHT OIL

When choosing oil, it's important to pick the right one. If you walk past the cheap cooking oils that are rich in omega-6s and go for oils that are rich in omega-3s instead, like, say, rapeseed or flaxseed oil, you've come a long way. Olive oil is also a good option because it contains a lot of wonderful anti-inflammatory polyphenols, as well as chlorophyll and vitamin E, which are two good safeguards against free radicals (and thus a good defense against inflammation).

The healthiest oils are often very heat sensitive, so make sure to only buy cold-pressed oils, which have not been heated during processing. Not only does the heat destroy delicate nutrients, it also creates chemical reactions that make otherwise healthy oil toxic. So never heat up any oils other than coconut oil, which has a high smoking point.

Speaking of coconut oil, it contains a specific saturated fat, MCT (which stands for Medium Chain Triglycerides, for those of you who enjoy taking notes). Simply, the body does not absorb MCT as easily as other fats. Also, coconut oil is antibacterial, which is, of course, a bonus.

Some good advice for anyone who likes saturated fat is to try coconut cream, which is easier for the body to absorb. This cream is rich in short- and medium-chain fatty acids.

HAVE WE OVERDONE OUR INCREASE IN FATS, MAYBE?

At around the time scientists figured out that it wasn't butter, cream, and cheese that made us fat, many people realized that one could eat large quantities of fat without putting on weight, as long as sugar and sugar-simulating foods were cut out. Excluding carbohydrates with high GI has shown to be an effective weapon against obesity, the greatest public health foe of our time. Many people have cured their type 2 diabetes by dietary changes alone, and without any medication.

Personally, we try to avoid sugar and sugar-simulating foods, but we are also a bit leery of gorging ourselves on all kinds of fat. Research shows that if you increase the amount of animal fats in your diet, it will lead (in as little as a few days) to an increase in the number of bad bacteria linked to illness and increased inflammation. Do you recall that fats can have different chain-lengths? Dairy and meat products are long-chained, which means they contain more than twelve carbon atoms. When we eat, the body absorbs nutrients through something called the hepatic portal vein and sends them on to the liver where they are quickly transformed into energy. Unfortunately, in the case of long-chain fats, their molecules are too big to make it through the portal vein, so the body must get its nutrients through the lymphatic system and the thoracic duct instead, and then let the fat spin around for hours in the blood, as if in a centrifuge, before the nutrients can at last reach the liver and be transformed into energy. *What's that? You think it's good that, for once, someone has the courage to do things their own way?* Well, you do have a point there. However, if we consume large amounts of long-chained fats, it becomes very stressful for the body.

Recall that we touched on endotoxin—a bacterial toxin—in the beginning of the book. Endotoxins are toxins produced by the bad bacteria that can fire up inflammation in the body. Studies show that the more animal fats one consumes, the more endotoxins the body creates. A meal containing a lot of fat can increase the level of endotoxins in the blood by as much as 50 percent.

A BRIEF SUMMARY

Fat is indispensible. You don't have to avoid saturated fat, but if you care about your intestinal flora, be cautious around the long-chained fats (in dairy and meat products). If you typically eat a lot of long-chained saturated fat, start by switching out some of it for its short-chained equivalent (cream and coconut cream).

We don't eat any more hydrogenated fats. Hydrogenated fats are the end result of an industrial process where polyunsaturated fatty acids have been turned into saturated fats to lengthen the shelf life of a product.

In the ideal world, the following applies:

1 Focus on good fats found in avocado, nuts, seeds, and good oils.
2 Ban hydrogenated fat from your diet.
3 Decrease your consumption of fish to a few times a week (consider that our oceans are overfished and otherwise not in great shape).

In the real world, we'll quickly turn the page for a shrimp treat—full of omega-3s and without even the slightest trace of hydrogenated fat.

FOOD PHARMACY'S SHRIMP FEAST

(makes 1 hearty bowl)

1 mango

1 avocado

A few cherry tomatoes

1 scallion

2 garlic cloves

½ chili

1 bunch fresh cilantro

Olive oil

Freshly squeezed lime juice

Salt and freshly ground black pepper

¾ lb (300 g) fresh shrimp, in the shell

We love shrimp. Back in the day we used to have them on toast with mayonnaise, but today we savor them with the world's loveliest avocado and mango salsa, lots of fresh cilantro, lime, and a bunch of anti-inflammatory omega-3s. Invite some friends over and get ready for praise. Curtsy and take a bow; but remain humble! The curtain falls.

Peel, remove the seeds, and dice the mango and avocado. Cut the tomatoes in half, chop the onion, peel and chop the garlic, slice the chili, and chop the cilantro. Mix all of it together. Season with olive oil and fresh lime juice. Add a bit of salt and pepper. Peel the shrimp and mix them carefully with the salsa. Serve as is, or in a salad with quinoa and leafy greens.

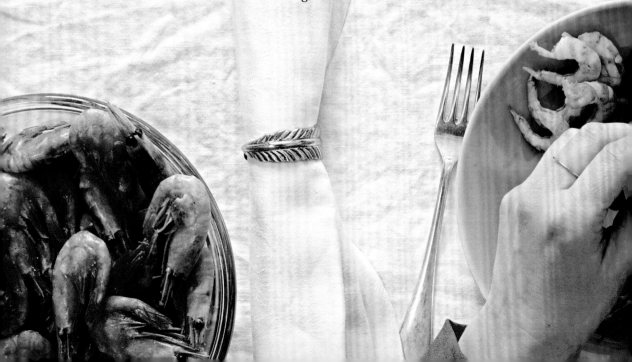

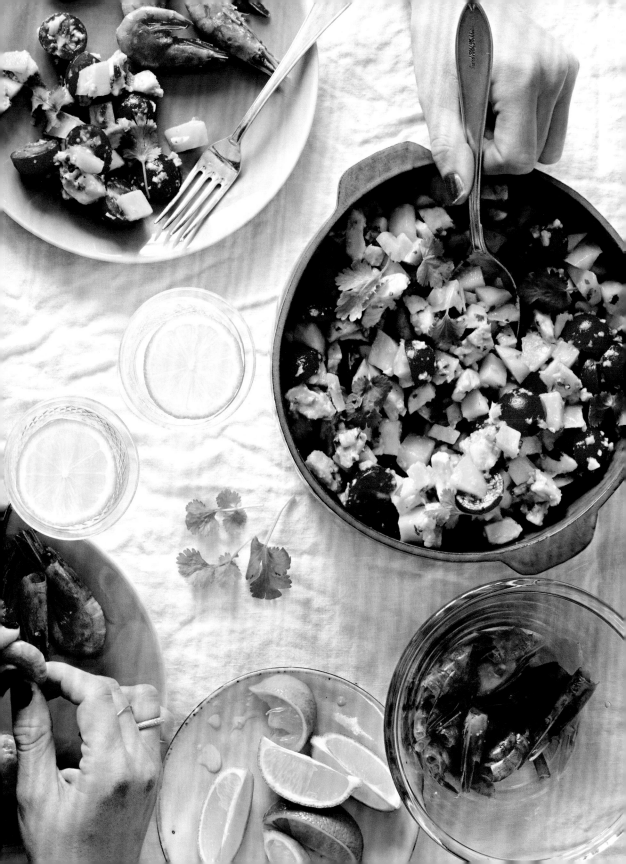

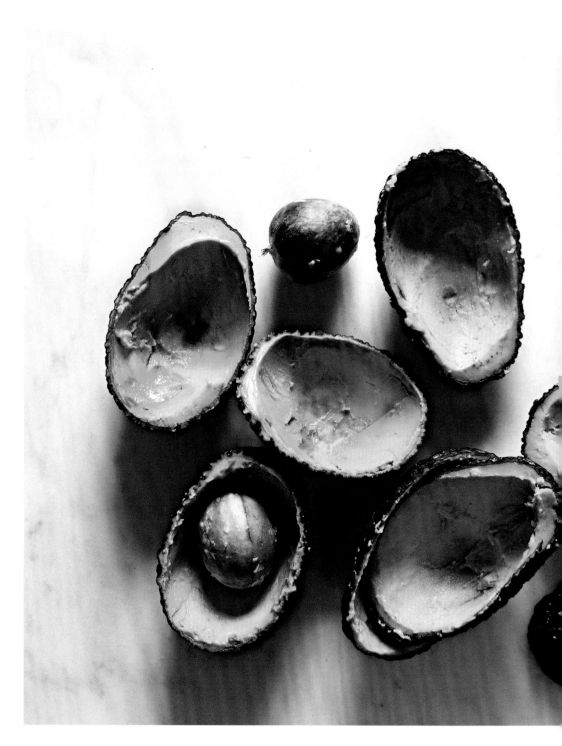

AVOCADO

Avocado has an almost supernatural ability to multitask and is good with everything—from salads to soup. Here's a tip for those whose children shun vegetables: add some avocado to colorful berries and turn it into a smoothie. Real fans insist that you can replace the butter in cookie dough with double the amount of avocado. We haven't tried that yet, but it's on our bucket list.

Avocados are one of our most nutrient-dense fruits—full of healthy fat, protein, and, let's not forget, fiber; if you want go all the way, you can eat the seed, too. The seed contains most of the avocado's antioxidants and a large part of its soluble fiber and healthy oils. If you feel that you may want to give it a try, cut the seed in half and then cut in half again; throw in one of the chunks when you're blending your soup or smoothie.

How do you know if you've used too much? Never fear: you'll taste it.

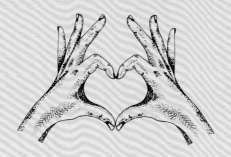

Boost Your Immune System

PROJECT: SAVE YOUR INTESTINAL FLORA

01.   Grab some paper and a pen.

02.   Write down what your Food Plate Model looks like in an ideal world. Are there many vegetables on it? Is there room for some meat and fish? Check out our commandments on page 6 if you don't know where to start.

03.   Now we have to deal with reality. Keep your ideal plate in mind when you plan your upcoming week's meals. Is most of what you eat something your good bacteria will enjoy? Can you swap one thing for a healthier option? Try to challenge yourself a bit more every week, and keep in mind that if you spoil Luke a little, you'll get it back ten fold (unlike when you spoil your children).

04.   Stay focused! A good way to do this is to buy your groceries online, that way you don't run the risk of letting those other things you shouldn't keep at home get in your shopping cart.

05. Clean out your pantry, and you'll decrease your chances of giving in to temptation. Dump everything that has no place around your intestinal flora in favor of things your good bacteria will like.

06. While you're at it, take this opportunity to clean out those secret treat stashes in the car, your desk drawer at work, and your purse, too. Load up on stuff that will keep cravings at bay and put an end to the impulse buys you make when your blood sugar takes a nosedive. As for us, we always carry a bag of nuts in our purses. It sounds pretty hard core, but trust us: it works.

07. It would be invaluable if you could get a buddy to join you in your quest to save the intestinal flora. You could give each other pep talks, and inspire and hug each other when things aren't going so great.

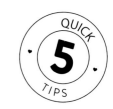

A brief summary about fats:

FIVE GREAT TIPS FOR THE INTESTINAL FLORA

01. Toss out all your cheap cooking oils and invest in cold-pressed olive, rapeseed, and coconut oil (the latter has highest smoking point).

02. An avocado a day makes Luke Skywalker happy.

03. Skip the hidden omega-6 villains like deep-fried foods, cookies and biscuits, stock cubes, prepackaged and processed foods, margarine, chips, and tortillas.

04. Consider adding a supplemental source of omega-3 to your diet, preferably krill oil.

05. Boost your meals with chia seeds or flaxseeds, and by all means enjoy a handful of walnuts daily.

LOWER THE HEAT

(save the nutrients and avoid the toxins created by heat)

When we got to know Professor Stig, we quickly found out that high cooking temperatures were probably not that good for the intestinal flora. That was sad for many reasons, but perhaps mostly because of crispbread. (If there's something we love, it's a slice of tasty crispbread covered in mashed avocado and coarse salt; reducing our consumption of this treat was not even an option.)

So we started baking our own crispbread instead, a version of it that intestinal flora can get behind. And, slowly but surely, it dawned on us that it's totally doable to bake and prepare food at slightly lower temperatures.

OUR HEAT CV (CURRICULUM VITAE)

We have always enjoyed eating warm food. And I mean really warm food—roasted, stir-fried, deep-fried, and grilled. We've loved crispy grilled chicken, thrown ourselves at the crustiest corner piece of the lasagna, and devoured blackened vegetables from the oven.

Our first grill was a regular charcoal grill. It stood at the back of the townhouse, and our neighbors were hanging in clusters over the potentilla to admire our new family member. Everything got cooked on the grill—hamburgers, chicken kebabs, corn on the cob, and marshmallows—and the food wasn't ready to eat until it had been thoroughly charred.

Our second grill was a gas grill that didn't get one break over an entire year. One New Year's Eve, we looked at our seafood and realized we could slap it on the grill. The result was burned lobster and champagne. That's the first and last time we tried that.

Our third and last grill was one of those small portable things you could bring along on a boat. We tied up our vessel to a suitably small sea boulder, jumped ashore, spread out our blankets, and threw our hot dogs on the grill. Success! When we returned to the city in the fall, the grill came home with us and was set out on the balcony. We continued to happily burn our meals at breakfast, lunch, and dinner until an upset neighbor knocked on the door. Naturally, we thought he was angry because his living room reeked of charred food, but imagine if he only had our intestinal flora's best interests at heart?

WHAT DO YOU MEAN, LOWER THE HEAT?

Most of us know that plant antioxidants are deactivated when they are heated up, and they don't need a lot of heat to do so (note to self: don't eat bell peppers in the sauna). It is said that the antioxidants begin to disappear at temperatures as low as 107.6°F (42°C), but in truth antioxidants in certain oils such as olive oil and rapeseed oil are destroyed around 86°F (30°C), which is why it's better to fry food in coconut oil, which can withstand higher temperatures.

When we first heard about the benefits of raw food, we thought it was because food loses its nutrients if you heat it up. *Ah yes, that makes sense*, we hummed, and added some extra carrot and celery sticks to our plate next to the charred chicken. Then we met Professor Stig, and we learned that there are other reasons for heating your food more gently, namely, toxins are created when very high heat is used in cooking. There are about a hundred varieties of these toxins, but the better known toxin among them is probably acrylamide. You'll find acrylamide in highly heated food.

In chemistry class at school, we learned that applying heat leads to synthetic processes that enable new substances to be created when two or more molecules form a bond. When food is exposed to temperatures of 176°F–212°F (80°C–100°C), its qualities are altered from its original form to become ever so slightly toxic. As you can see on page 143, a dramatic change occurs at over 320°F (160°C). The most common reaction is when food is cooked to the point where a protein molecule bonds with a sugar molecule. This is called *glycation*, and the end products are called *advanced glycation products* (AGE). It's also common for a protein to bond with a fat, which is called *lipoxidation*, and the end products are called *advanced lipoxidantion products* (ALE).

Professor Stig says that to eat AGE and ALE is like smoking with your stomach. AGE and ALE stoke inflammation in the body and contribute to chronic inflammation and chronic illnesses. Luke sinks into a dark pit of despair. Darth throws up a high-five.

The worst villains in ALE and AGE are French fries and dark-roasted coffee, as well as bread, biscuits, and cookies that have been baked, deep-fried, or roasted. Following is a list of a few obvious bad guys that contain larger amounts of AGE and ALE.

Instant milk powder
- Ice cream
- Infant formula and instant oatmeal

Grain products
- Cookies
- Toast
- Rusks (twice-baked bread)
- Crispbread
- Breakfast cereal

Miscellaneous products
- Coffee (especially dark roast)
- Fast foods like pizza, nachos, and tacos
- Sweet whey cheese and sweet whey cheese spread
- Roasted nuts
- Dark soy sauce

SCIENCE FOR YOU

Most known plant antioxidants are rendered inactive if heated to between 107.6°F and 212°F (42°C and 100°C).

Lina is struggling to free a doggie-doo bag from her pocket.

– No kidding—milk powder! Isn't that the basic ingredient in children's formula?

– Oh my God, total anxiety attack. My children drank huge amounts of formula.

– Mine too!

Both glance at Pyret, who is sniffing intensely at something in a flowerbed.

– Don't you remember how we used to sit with our bottles of formula at preschool? It was so much more convenient to bring along a carton of formula instead of mashing up avocado and banana and lightly cooked vegetables.

– Well, at that time our priority was on how much sleep we could get at night and what brand of crib was best. We didn't know that intestinal flora is especially sensitive in a baby's first years, a time when the immune system matures.

A long silence follows. It looks like Pyret has picked up a scent.

Fig. #7

ACRYLAMIDE VALUES IN OVEN-BAKED FRENCH FRIES
(Source: Tareke C et al J. Agric. FoodChem. 2002;50:4998-5006)

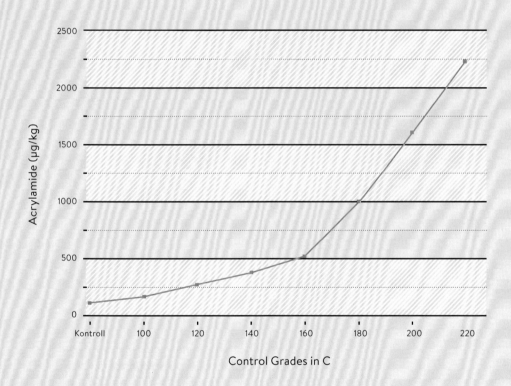

– Why didn't they warn us about this at the children's clinic?

– Not a clue. But I just read an article that describes brilliantly how anyone on Earth could ever have imagined that formula—a mix of flour, dried milk, and some added nutrients—would be better for toddlers than home-prepped meals.

– It's crazy. I feel like I've been totally conned. Sorry, hang on . . . Pyret, Pyret, come back!

Pyret notices an elegant standard poodle on the other side of the park and takes off.

DOES THIS MEAN I HAVE TO BECOME A RAW-FOODER NOW?

Not at all. Of course, your good bacteria will be delighted to encounter some raw vegetables, but it's a fact that you'll be heading in the right direction if you lower your oven's temperature considerably, and if you steam and simmer your food instead of frying and grilling it to a crisp.

The raw-food kitchen sets the limit at 107.6°F (42°C) and Professor Stig prefers his at 176°F (80°C). It may sound difficult the first time you cook like this, but the truth is that fish, poultry, and meat only gets more tender and tasty when cooked at a lower heat. It's a bit trickier with bread, which unfortunately requires a higher inner cooking temperature, but our prescription crispbread on the next page is fully baked at 158°F (70°C).

We totally get it if you feel that it's a lot of work to change the temperature, but if you take that feeling, subtract it by ten, then divide that by four, you'll see the true effort it'll take. It's not very hard at all. We still make the same kind of foods as before, the only difference being that we prefer to use the oven instead of the stovetop.

Then there are vegetables that benefit from being heated. Just when we grasped the idea that antioxidant levels go down when heated, we find out that this doesn't hold true for tomatoes. Tomatoes contain an antioxidant called *lycopene,* and unlike other antioxidants lycopene loves heat so much that it actually increases when tomatoes are heated up and cooked.

Thus, a cooked tomato sauce will provide more lycopene than a raw tomato salsa. You'll also find lycopene in apricots, ruby grapefruit, watermelon, pink guava, papaya, red bell peppers, hawthorn, goji berries, and rose hips . . . just so you know.

SO WHAT DO WE DO NOW?

As we mentioned, we've always liked warm food, but when we realized that the nutrients in vegetables are lost if we heat them, and that blackened pieces of lasagna feed Darth's army, we had to rethink our habits a bit.

In the ideal world the following rules apply:
1 Always try to avoid intense heat, as in grilling and sautéing.
2 Try to keep the oven's heat at under 212°F (100°C), even when preparing fish, poultry, and meat dishes.
3 As most of us know, poultry needs to reach an inner temperature of at least 158°F (70°C). Meat, however, only needs heat between 122°F (50°C) for rare and 212°F (70°C) for well done; most fish will be at its best around 133°F (56°C).

Increasing the temperature from 212°F (100°C) to 248°F (120°C) creates especially carcinogenic chemicals called heterocyclic amines.

And in the real world we'll do as we usually do: as best we can. The most important thing for us is that food retains as much of its nutritional value as possible, and we obviously want to avoid heat-generated toxins. These changes didn't really spring up overnight, and both of us still keep a frying pan around to make crepes (don't tell Stig), but in fact we do make them less and less.

Starting to eat large amounts of raw vegetables wasn't really a chore for us, but we still liked warm food a little too much to give it up entirely. It was no big deal to lower the heat a few notches, but eating everything cold and never cooking again was a bit too extreme. So we developed our very own cooking technique. You could say that we've become food magicians of a sort in how we mix warm and cold food. Here are our best tips; there are, of course, endless variations on these themes.

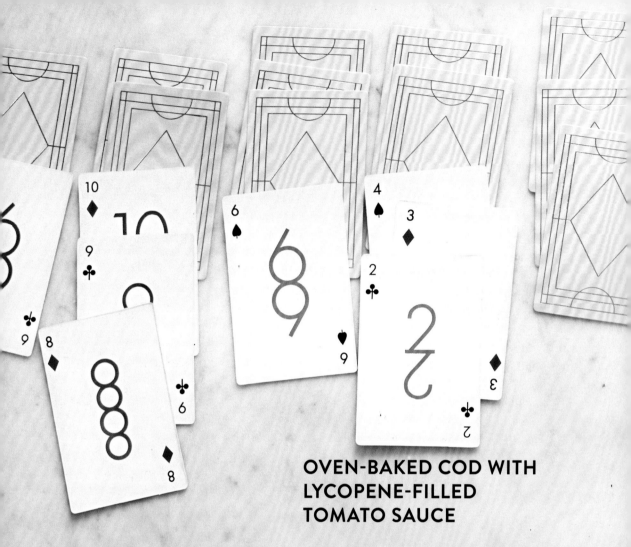

OVEN-BAKED COD WITH LYCOPENE-FILLED TOMATO SAUCE

⁴/₅ lb (400 g) frozen cod

1 yellow onion, peeled

2 garlic cloves, peeled

1¹/₅ lb (500 g) crushed tomatoes

One piece fresh ginger, finely grated

1 tbsp stock powder

1 tbsp coconut oil

Salt and freshly ground black pepper

Parsley

This cod is prepared at a lower temperature than usual, which is why cooking time is slightly longer. To keep yourself busy while you wait: play solitaire, teach yourself to become an astronaut, learn a new language.

The sauce can be made in the blink of an eye: chop everything coarsely and blend for 30 seconds. Defrost the fish and place it in an ovenproof dish; pour the tomato sauce over and sprinkle with parsley. Place the dish in a 70°C (158°F) oven (if you have a digital thermometer, set it to 132°F [56°C]). Cook for about 1 hour. Serve the fish with quinoa or sorghum grains drizzled with some coconut oil, and the kids' favorite vegetables.

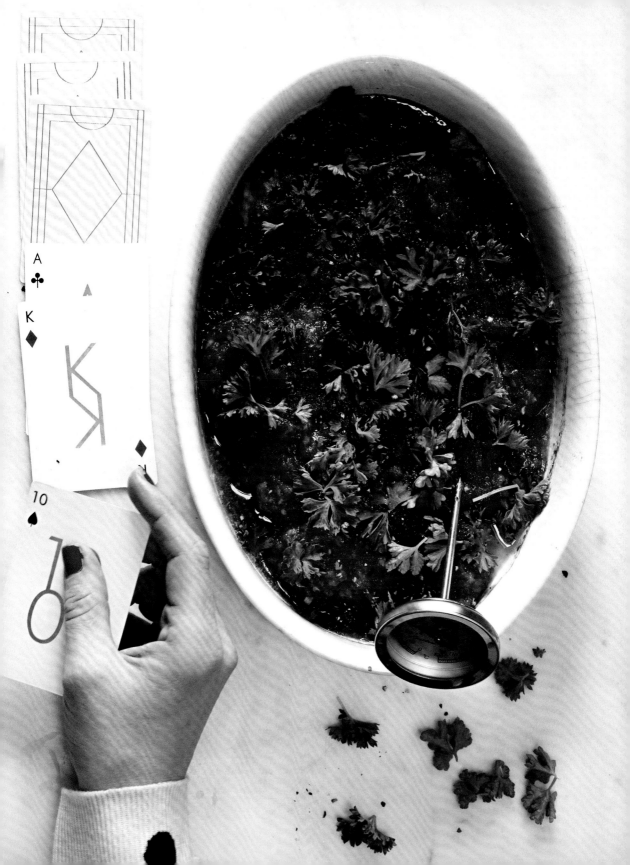

You may stop reading now, Gordon Ramsay; for the rest of you everyday cooks out there, here are some tips.

Magic trick #1
We boil lentils in stock and let them cool down a little. We transfer them to a blender, mix them with a lot of raw vegetables, and press the Start button. End result: warm lentil soup with raw vegetables.

Magic trick #2
We oven-bake cod at a low temperature with tomatoes, which we know become more nutritious with heat. We serve the fish with a mound of cold potato salad. End result: warm cod with vegetables.

Magic trick #3
Cook sorghum grains in boiling water. Pour away the water and mix the grains with raw vegetables, oil, salt, nuts, pepper, and lots of wonderful herbs. End result: warm "risotto" (come on, use your imagination) and raw vegetables.

To appreciate using less heat fully, you'll have to try it yourself. Start with the above recipes or attempt your own variations. You can still eat warm food, but the heat you use should be gentle. You'll find that you won't be heating some of the dishes you used to warm up.

And in the meantime, you'll get a lot of stuff done while the food is taking its own sweet time in the oven. For instance, the crispbread that's coming up can't be made in just 25 minutes. The advantage is that you now have time for other things while you wait. Set a bowl with a few different vegetables on the table, and snack on some antioxidants. Or pair up your socks in the laundry pile. Everybody who has attempted this knows that this task has no time limit.

Heating in the microwave creates AGE and ALE, too.

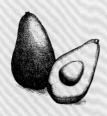

A SMALL-ISH LIST OF SUBSTITUTIONS

Butter:	Avocado, nut butters
Milk:	Almond, nut, and oat milk
Cream:	Coconut milk and cream, oat cream
Breakfast flakes:	Unsweetened muesli or granola, chia seed pudding
Iceberg lettuce:	Spinach, kale, arugula, romaine lettuce
Store-bought juice:	Homemade smoothie
Pasta:	Bean noodles, spiralized carrots or zucchini, kelp noodles
Rice:	Sorghum grains, quinoa, buckwheat
Oil:	Cold-pressed coconut oil, rapeseed or olive oil
White sugar:	Fruit, berries

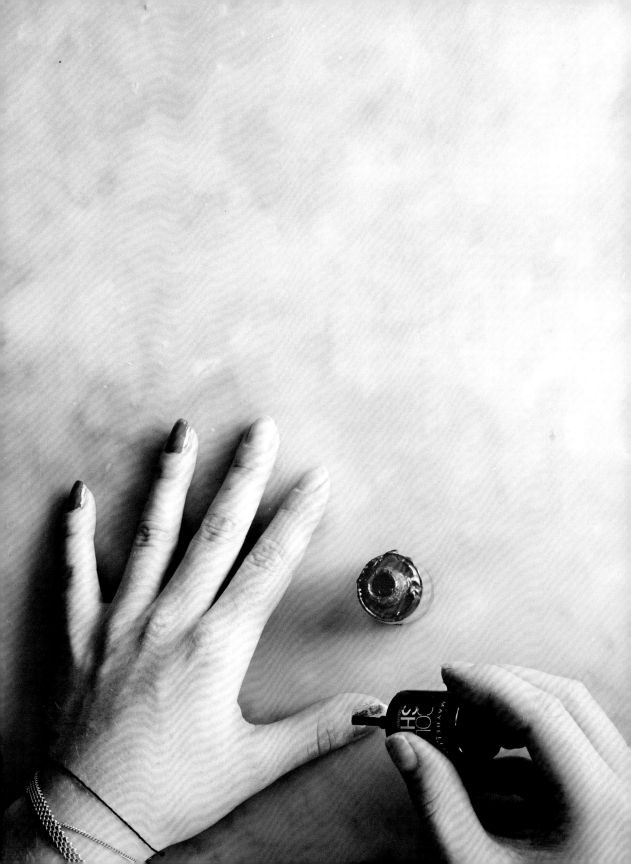

CRISPBREAD WORTH WAITING FOR

(makes one baking sheet full)

²/₅ cup (100 ml) sorghum flour

²/₅ cup (100 ml) rolled oats

²/₅ cup (100 ml) sunflower seeds

²/₅ cup (100 ml) sesame seeds

¹/₅ cup (50 ml)) pumpkin seeds

¹/₅ cup (50 ml) flaxseeds

1 tsp cumin powder

½ tsp salt

¹/₅ cup (50 ml) rapeseed oil

⁴/₅ cup (200 ml) boiling water

Stig's wife, Marianne, shared this recipe with us. Upon reflection, maybe we shouldn't call it crispbread, as the texture is a bit more on the crumbly side. But crumbly bread sounds a bit weird, doesn't it? In any case, whatever you decide to call it, it's delicious.

Preheat the oven to no higher than 160°F (71°C). Mix everything together and transfer onto a sheet of parchment paper. Place another piece of parchment paper on top of the dough and press it out with your hands or a rolling pin (make sure you don't make it too thin, or it will crack very easily). Remove the top sheet of paper and, if you want, draw squares on the dough with a ruler. Sprinkle some sea salt flakes over the dough and put it in the oven. Keep the oven door open a little bit to let the steam escape, and try to be patient for at least 2 hours. Let the bread cool off and spread it with your choice of toppings.

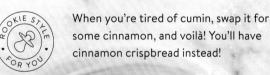

When you're tired of cumin, swap it for some cinnamon, and voilà! You'll have cinnamon crispbread instead!

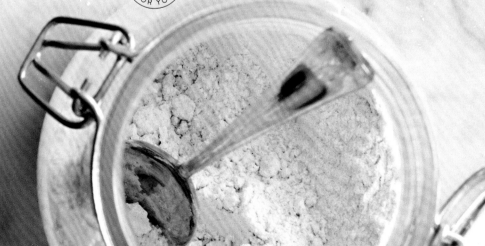

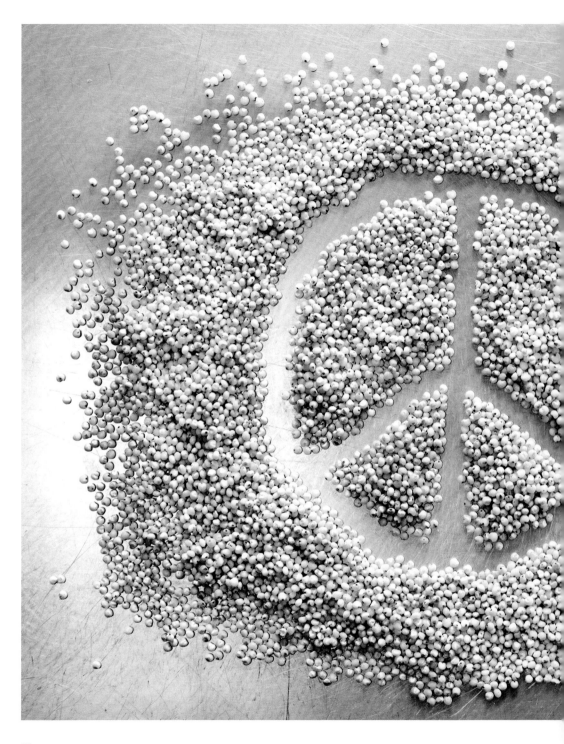

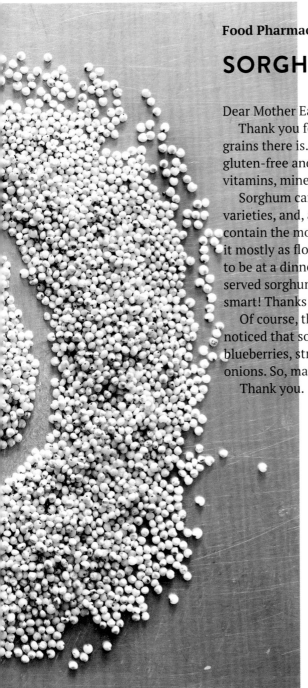

SORGHUM

Dear Mother Earth.

Thank you for sorghum—one of the most nutritious grains there is. Thank you for making it naturally gluten-free and for imparting it with lots of wholesome vitamins, minerals, and antioxidants.

Sorghum can come in black, red, and brown varieties, and, as usual, the most colorful grains contain the most antioxidants. This past year, we used it mostly as flour when we've baked, but we happened to be at a dinner party recently where the hostess served sorghum to the kids instead of rice. That's really smart! Thanks for that tip!

Of course, this is not a competition, but we have noticed that sorghum contains more antioxidants than blueberries, strawberries, plums, broccoli, carrots, and onions. So, many thanks for that, too.

Thank you.

A brief summary about temperatures:

FIVE TIPS ON COOKING TEMPERATURES FOR THE INTESTINAL FLORA

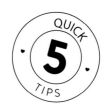

01. Do you love frying? Fine, but lower the heat by a few notches if you do. Let it take a little longer to cook. Use coconut oil, which has a higher smoking point than olive oil and rapeseed oil.

02. Start using the oven more often and the frying pan less. The things we fry—fish, meat, and vegetables—cook just as well in the oven.

03. As for vegetables, eat them raw if you wish to maximize their nutrients.

04. Bake your own bread and crispbread.

05. Dare to try new recipes that don't require an oven.

Prescription #6

GIVE YOUR BODY A CHANCE TO REBOOT NOW AND THEN

(using periodic/intermittent fasting)

We drink a lot of tea. In Plato's ideal world we would each be sitting in a comfy chair, listening to the radio, and reading Maya Angelou, but unfortunately in the real world we get interrupted. One child is hell-bent on killing his or her sibling, or does a cartwheel right into the bookcase, so the tea has time to go cold while we call an ambulance. That's when we realized we could pour it into our smoothie. In the ideal world we skip breakfast, but when the real world becomes too challenging we fix things with the smoothie from this chapter. It's almost ideal, because the body doesn't absorb raw vegetables until they've reached the colon anyway, so you can eat a little earlier than usual but still allow the organ rest and detox for another two to three more hours. If that isn't smart, what is?

OUR BREAKFAST CV (CURRICULUM VITAE)

One little snag you can hit when writing a book with another person is that it can give the impression that the authors are joined at the hip—when going to the store, picking up the kids, or going to the bathroom. That's why we're letting you know right now that when it comes to breakfast, we are as different as Tom and Jerry.

There are two sorts of people in this world:

1 Morning people
2 People who want to shoot morning people.

Lina is a person who sleeps with her finger on the trigger. And she wakes up ravenous. In the past, breakfast was the only thing that got her out of bed in the morning. Now, when she doesn't eat breakfast, coffee is the only thing that gets her up and about. Can you imagine if she were to quit drinking coffee? We would have to work from our beds.

Mia, however, is fully awake before the alarm goes off. She is in her prime in the morning, AM being the time of day when everything is possible and fun. Things go steadily south from then on: she feels more and more tired and gets gradually hungrier; by 9 p.m. she'll eat anything, whether her intestinal flora reacts or not.

This explains why it wasn't a great day for any of us when Professor Stig dropped the bomb and said we would feel much better if we skipped both breakfast and dinner.

"BREAKFAST IS OUR LEAST IMPORTANT MEAL"

It all started when we read an article Professor Stig had written about gluttony. Two points made us sit up and pay attention, namely 1) rates of sickness skyrocket over Christmas and New Year because we eat so much, and 2) Stig had the audacity to claim that breakfast was the least important meal of the day.

Let's back up a bit.

1 Acute illness, strokes, and heart attacks in particular often occur in concurrence with large meals and big holidays. At Christmas and New Year, the prevalence of illness and mortality hits the roof, and hospital emergency departments are filled to capacity. The burden is too great for the body's organs to be on the receiving end of such large quantities of sugar, sugar-simulating foods, and fat—we gorge over the holidays and our bodies simply can't handle it. Our bodies do not give us a free pass just because it's the weekend or Christmas.

2 Skip breakfast. What the . . . ? Surely everybody knows that breakfast is the most important meal of the day? *Nope*, says Professor Stig, calmly and deliberately, *because if you eat breakfast and dinner every day, your organs never have a chance to rest.*

As it turns out, Stig has been fasting every day now for years. He sets aside a few hours during which he eats no food so that his organs can rest for most of the day. We have seen different versions of this method and haven't found any strict guidelines, but the ideal world promotes a ratio of 18:6 or 16:8 (you fast for 18 or 16 hours and eat over a period of 6 or 8 hours). During the fast you can only drink water, coffee, or tea, i.e., noncalorific drinks.

PERIODIC/INTERMITTENT FASTING

It's no accident that this prescription comes last in the book. It's incredibly important to know how to put together a nourishing meal before you start practicing intermittent fasting. The whole point of fasting is to give the cells an opportunity to recover and give them time to function without hindrance. The last food we consume before fasting should be like an elaborate tasting menu for Luke and his army—nutrient-dense food full of fiber that gives the bacteria a chance to grow and multiply. If the day's meals tend toward macaroni, bologna, pizza, and pastry for dessert, you're feeding Darth Vader's army instead and leaving the good bacteria to starve. If this is the case, then you should hold off on fasting and concentrate on getting started on the rest of the program first.

Regardless of what you choose to do, intermittent fasting is one of the best and cheapest methods to deal with inflammation, according to many scientists. New research also shows that intermittent fasting might be an effective tool in halting the activation of undesirable genes, thus being a practical example of how you can personally benefit from epigenetics and counteract unwanted genetic triggers. In fact, several scientists practice periodic fasting themselves. This is not a weight loss technique, but rather a way of life that can provide many health advantages (however, we do not recommend that you fast if you are a child, pregnant, or nursing, or if you suffer from any type of eating disorder).

A green smoothie is not absorbed by the body until two to three hours after ingestion, which means that the organs' time of rest and detox is extended by two hours. That's how long it takes the vegetables to reach the beneficial bacteria—the only ones that can deal with this kind of food.

CALORIC RESTRICTION

As far back as 2,000 BC, i.e., around the time the books of Moses were written, the story was told of how Moses fasted in the desert for forty days. Gluttony was pegged as one of the seven deadly sins, and the Old Testament upheld moderation as a virtue. Fasting is a feature of all major religions, the best known religious event being Ramadan, the Muslim month of fasting.

Science caught up with this concept in the twentieth century, and in the mid-'80s *calorie restriction* (CR), where you only eat two-thirds of your hypothetical daily caloric requirements, was shown to have important health effects on all the animals studied. Test subjects had up to twice the life expectancy and significantly lower rates of illness, and they showed considerable delays in the manifestation of chronic illness. Even though studies on human subjects are still nowhere near as advanced as we'd like, many scientists all over the world report important progress when humans are asked to restrict their calories. As long as they receive enough of all necessary nutrients, they lessen their risk of suffering from diabetes, cardiovascular disease, and cancer, compared to people who do not practice fasting.

Lately, scientists have begun to express further interest in intermittent fasting and its proven health benefits. They have concluded that these benefits are more or less identical to those derived by calorie restriction. When you fast in the short-term, your body does everything to protect your cells from injury, which lowers blood pressure and produces better insulin sensitivity. This is how the body halts inflammation and aging. If you turn the equation around, the opposite holds true: a constant, high intake of calories makes the body increase its rate of cell division, which in turn leads to unnecessary premature aging.

To experience the full benefits of CR (calorie restriction), you should reduce the amount of protein you eat, especially the intake of the amino acid methionine, which is plentiful in animal products.

ARE YOU AWARE THAT YOU HAVE A FAT SWITCH?

There are three ways that nutrients can be stored in the body:
1 As sugar, in the liver and muscles, called *glycogen*. The storage limit for that is 800 calories.
2 As abdominal fat. Our ancestors stored about 500 calories this way, but today there are examples of people who have stored up to 54,000 calories (13.22 lb / 6 kg).
3 As subcutaneous fat. This type of fat isn't as dangerous as abdominal fat, but it's still linked to poor health and chronic illness. Subcutaneous fat hoards a lot of junk like toxins, hormones, drugs, bacterial debris, and bacterial toxins.

At the risk of oversimplifying things a little, you could say that the body prefers to run on sugar (glucose), but if you don't fill up on new food when sugar runs low, it forces the body to turn on the "fat switch" and start burning fat instead. There are many signs that fat burning doesn't start in earnest until glucose stores

Fig. #8

DAILY FASTING AND HEALTH

(Source: Hatori M et al Cell Metabolism 2012; 15: 848–860)

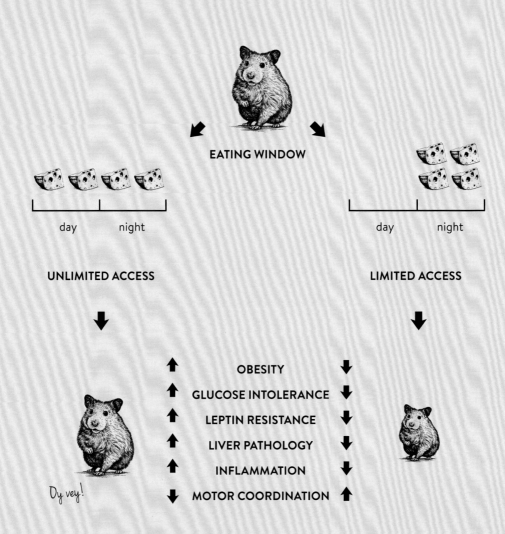

are empty. And why is it good to burn fat? Well, among other things, the body has a bad habit of using fat as a temporary garbage bin, where it stores everything from drug residue, bacteria, debris, and environmental toxins. If you force your body into burning fat, you'll get rid of those toxins at the same time.

Let's do some arithmetic here:
Pretend that you eat your last meal of the day at 6 p.m., and that it contains about 800 calories. If you read or watch TV, you'll burn about 85 calories per hour, which means that you'll have used up about half of those 800 calories by the time you're tucked into bed by 10:30 or 11 p.m. While you're sleeping, your calorie burn goes down to about 65 calories per hour, which means the calories you ate at last night's dinner are totally spent by morning. Click. What's that sound? Ah, that's the fat switch that turned itself on, which means the body will now start burning fat instead of calories. For this to benefit you, you should leave your body alone for about six hours (which equals approximately 500–600 calories in body fat) of this process.

A recent study using mice illustrates the benefits brought on by intermittent fasting. The mice were divided into two groups and given exactly the same amount of calories of food, but with one single difference—one group of mice could eat whenever they wanted, while the other group could only eat over a period of less than half of 24 hours.

Look at the picture on p. 160: The animals that had free access to food over the 24-hour period got rounder and rounder, and sicker and sicker, while the other group, which went through a daily period of fasting, became leaner and healthier, even though they were ingesting the same amount of calories. The liver of the mice that could eat at will took a particularly hard hit. The mice even had trouble handling sugar (their glucose tolerance decreased) and their muscle function and satiety hormone became blunted (this is called leptin resistance in medical terminology). Leptin resistance stops the body's satiety signal—the messenger to the brain that tells us to stop eating after we've consumed enough food—from working, the effect being that we continue to eat more than we need.

FASTING SMOOTHIE FOR THE REAL WORLD

(makes one large cup)

1 handful leafy greens

²/₅ cup (100 ml) blueberries

½ avocado

Few drops freshly squeezed lemon juice

5 fresh mint leaves

1¹/₅ cups (300 ml) cold green tea

Take a seat in your comfiest chair, and enjoy this smoothie until your kids start running wild again (20 seconds, max).

Mix everything and pour into two large glasses.

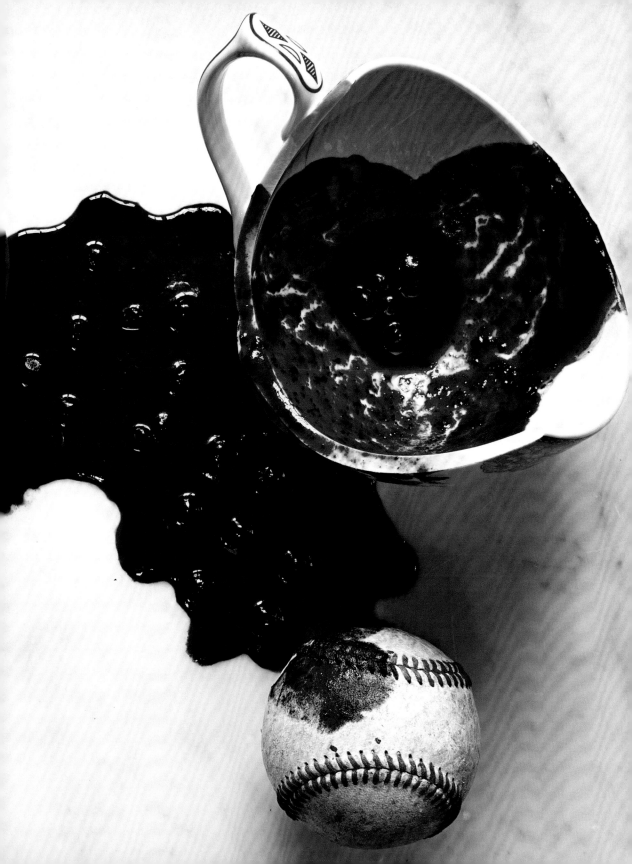

Lina and Mia are in the stables. Mia is carefully measuring Juventus's food into a bowl.

– When you do this for animals, nobody questions it.

Lina grooms Yen.

– I know, right? I'm always telling the kids that Pyret will get sick if they give her more food than her little portions in the morning and at night. It's the same with horses. Imagine if we stuffed them with crispbread, carrots, and lumps of sugar all the time.

Juventus snorts.

– Well, it applies to a lot of other things we've mentioned in the book, too. Who would ever get the idea to give Pyret anything other than water on Saturdays, just because it happens to be the weekend? It's the pet owner's job to make sure that his or her pet's diet is healthy. It seems obvious, but if you're a mom who keeps an eye on what her kids eat, you're kind of automatically tagged as boring and un-fun.

Mia and Lina lead their horses out into the field. The bumblebees buzz and the sheep bleat. The two women hop onto their horses and ride bareback into the woods.

THE BLUE ZONES

When Belgian scientist Michel Poulain and his Italian colleague Gianni Pes discovered that a high percentage of centenarians hailed from the mountain regions of Sardinia, they quickly circled the area on the map with a blue pen. That's the origin of the term "blue zone," and since then several other areas that have atypical numbers of centenarians have been circled in, among them Okinawa in Japan and the Nicoya peninsula in Costa Rica. Naturally, there are some similarities between them, but it isn't as simple as these blue zone populations eating identical things. Some eat fish but never meat; others never eat fish but do eat bread. The amount of meat on their plates may vary, but vegetables are everywhere in large varieties—especially green leafy vegetables and legumes—and are all completely sugar-free and without additives.

It would be a lie to suggest that these inhabitants practiced intermittent fasting, but you could say that they practice short-term fasting of a sort every day. Historically, access to food has been a bit more limited in blue zones, which means that the inhabitants of those regions are used to eating less in general. Also, a common thread among them is eating a light breakfast and dinner, and making lunch their day's main meal. By not consuming a bigger meal at night, they get to rest their stomach almost 12 hours out of the day's 24.

People living in the blue zones survive on an average of 1,700 to 1,800 calories per day, even though they work long hours in their fields. Compare these numbers to what the USDA recommends: 1,600–2,400 calories for women and 2,000–3,000 calories for men. In the same way that there is a common trait among people living in the blue zones—they enjoy long life spans—there is also a common trait among the people who live in areas with high calorie intake: they tend to age prematurely, suffer from high inflammatory stress in the body, and to a large extent are beset by more chronic disease than ever before in history. In Okinawa, an island off the coast of Japan and one of the blue zones, they have a saying: "*Hara hachi bu*," meaning there should always be a small empty space left in your belly after you've eaten. In other words, don't stuff yourself. This is a given in Okinawa and a somewhat empty belly isn't considered a problem, but that might also have something to do with the fact that they eat slowly. That's another reason to not scarf your food down. Otherwise, not only will you become uncomfortably full but you will also eat way more than is necessary.

DON'T YOU GET HUNGRY WHEN YOU FAST?

Encouraged by Professor Stig and his talk of the fat switch and the blue zones, we finally decided to give intermittent fasting a try. We were enticed by the fact that we could eat exactly the same as before, if we only moved breakfast a few hours out, and quit eating an hour or so earlier at night, while reaping tons of health benefits.

It's worth a try, we thought.

We planned to do it for one week. Well, you can already predict the challenges we faced: Lina, who wakes up hungry as a wolf each morning, had great trouble skipping breakfast; Mia, who is soft as a lamb until the early afternoon, experienced great stress in the evening. As the sun disappeared behind the horizon, her stomach began complaining so loudly that the neighbors called the police. The police: "Can you turn it down?" Mia: "Sorry, that was just my belly growling."

But then something quite unexpected happened: We felt more alert. Intermittent fasting makes you feel intensely awake and focused. When we did some research on this, we learned that it had a biological explanation: intermittent fasting makes you concentrate because the brain boosts its growth factor, which in turn produces synapses and helps protect the brain cells. It's basically the result of evolution: when times were hard and food scarce, it was important to focus and remember where we found food the last time, for example, or figure out how to satisfy our immediate needs. If we became weak and tired at those times, and simply laid down on the ground, the entire human race would have died out.

Well, at least we felt more alert.

IT'S OKAY TO ONLY DO THIS THREE DAYS A WEEK

Then we hit another snag. Question: How can you be part of a social life when you fast? Answer: You don't.

Very few friends are going to want to have dinner with you at 5:30 p.m. on a Friday night, and your family will get fed up real quick if you turn up to weekend brunch only to sip your green tea. So, we were ecstatic to learn that it's enough to do intermittent fasting a few times a week. It delivers the same measurable effects as calorie restriction, provided you follow a sound diet the rest of the time. Perhaps it seems a bit unnatural to eat more on some days and less on others, but again, if we glance in the rearview mirror and look at how our ancestors did things, we'll see that they also ate very irregularly because their access to resources varied tremendously.

This worked perfectly for us.

In the ideal world we do the following:

1 Two to seven days a week, we don't consume anything besides liquids for at least 16 hours; eat as you would the rest of the time.
2 Make sure that the main meal is eaten at the same time each day.
3 Make sure your meals are nutrient-dense so you get everything you need.

How you set up your fasting plan is totally up to you and according to your real world. Many healthy and long-living groups of people eat an early dinner around 4 p.m. and then a light breakfast, while others make lunch their principal meal. One of the most eminent researchers in this field practices intermittent fasting two to three times a week—he skips breakfast and lunch, breaking his fast with some fruit in the early afternoon, and then enjoys dinner with his family. Research has shown that the main meal is almost as important as daylight is for guiding our hormonal clock. Also, keep in mind that anyone who eats little needs to eat especially well to make sure they get enough vitamins, minerals, and other nutrients. If you only eat boozy chocolates and quick carbohydrates, you'd be better off gaining control of your eating habits, and proceeding from there to fasting. But you know by now how to eat in order to live without inflammation. You will have soon read an entire book on the subject here.

Listen up now, because this is important: Always listen to your body, and proceed slowly. If your normal eating window has been 6 a.m. to 10 p.m. up until now, then it's probably best not to go right in to a 16:8 schedule. Maybe you could start with 14:1 instead, otherwise you may quit fasting right away. Take baby steps!

ANYONE CAN FAST

Well, we had to get here eventually—to the end of this book. You have now received six prescriptions, which we hope will be a great start to your anti-inflammatory journey.

Here are two things we know for sure:

1 We will miss you. Promise you'll check in on our blog ten times a day.
2 We all face different obstacles.

Even the two of us have faced completely different challenges. It might be difficult to imagine, but it wasn't all that long ago that Mia was the champion of candy eating—the bag of sweets was usually empty before she even got into the movie theater. And then we have Lina, with her weird cravings for sugar-simulating food, also difficult to fathom today.

Maybe you've got totally different issues and excuses. You've probably already dreamt up thousands of reasons why it's not a good idea to avoid all sugar-simulating food at this very moment; or why you can't start buying organic vegetables until you've been given that salary raise; or why you can't sell your deep-fryer on Craigslist until summer's over.

And all those things are probably true. Maybe you should wait for that raise. But it doesn't matter who you are, where you live, and how you work; there is one thing that no excuse in the world can overpower: intermittent fasting. It's simple, it's affordable, it requires no extra time, it accommodates allergies, you don't have to buy anything, and it works wherever you are in the world. Amen.

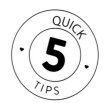

A brief summary about intermittent fasting:

FIVE FASTING TIPS FOR THE INTESTINAL FLORA

01. We believe that you should ease into it at the beginning, and maybe start by skipping breakfast or your evening sandwich.

02. Or, maybe you could eat breakfast an hour or two later, or alternatively eat your last meal of the day an hour earlier.

03. Start by implementing changes one or two days per week.

04. If you don't want to skip breakfast, sip a green drink in the morning—as we've already mentioned, raw and green hardly taxes the digestive system in the first few hours since it needs to travel all the way down to the colon's bacteria. Consequently, you can eat a little earlier than usual, and still let your organs' rest continue undisturbed for another two to three hours after breakfast.

05. Drink gallons of tea during the fasting hours.

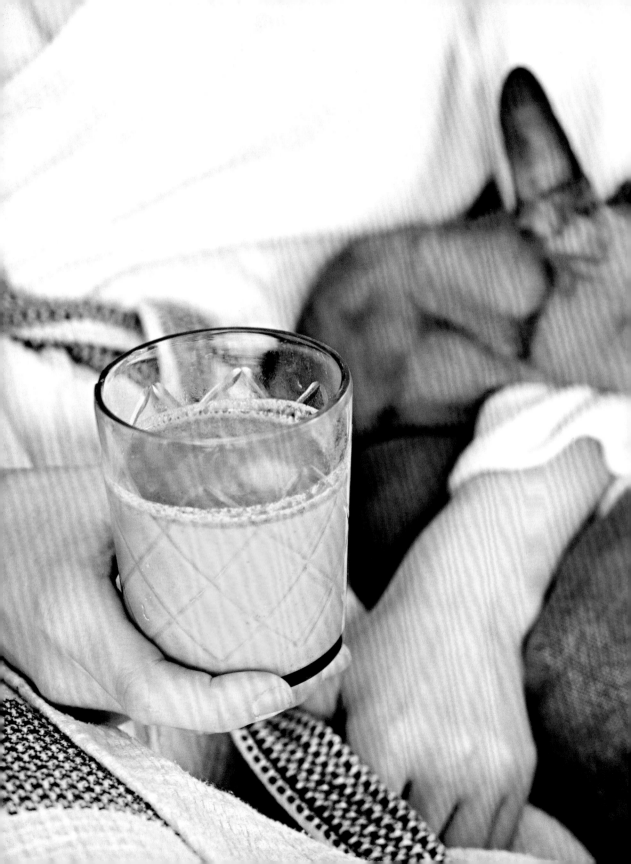

GOLDEN ANTI-INFLAMMATORY MILK

(makes 2 glasses)

2¼ cups (500 ml) almond or oat milk

1 tbsp ground turmeric

1 tsp ground cinnamon

1 tsp ground cardamom

⅕ tsp (1 ml) vanilla powder

1 tsp black pepper

1 tbsp coconut oil

1 tbsp honey

This is a gentler version of Professor Stig's shot of turmeric (page 14). It's perfect if you have tried the shot but think it's too intense. They say that this golden milk works well as a sleeping aid, but it's also good at any hour of the day.

Heat the milk until it's lukewarm. Whisk in the rest of the ingredients and drink the milk immediately. Nighty night!

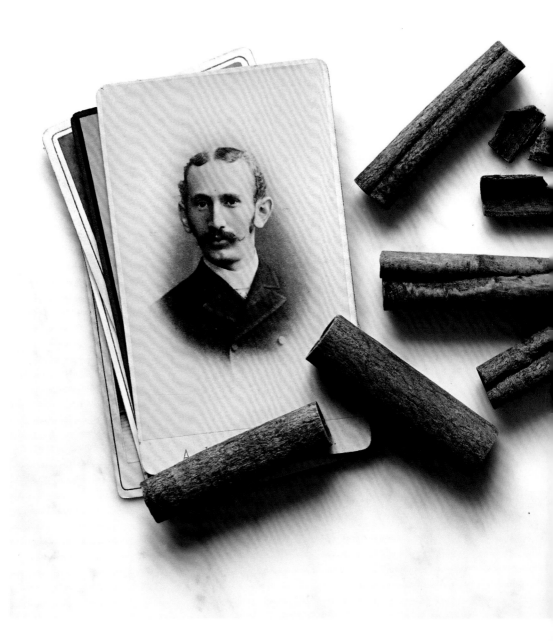

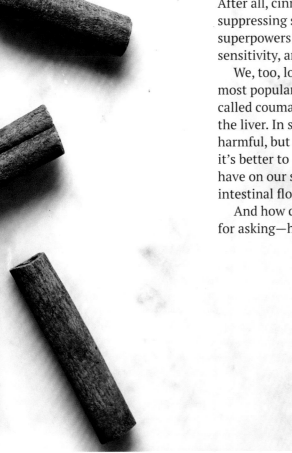

CINNAMON

Let us tell you about Hugo Cinnamon. Hugo Cinnamon was Lina's great-great-uncle. His real last name was Lindgren, but everyone soon forgot that as soon as he started sprinkling cinnamon over anything edible that came his way. Hugo Cinnamon really loved cinnamon. Back in the day, he was considered a bit loopy because he sprinkled cinnamon on his fish, meat, and eggs, but today we know he was doing the right thing. After all, cinnamon is one of the most inflammation-suppressing spices in the spice rack, and it also has superpowers to lower blood fats, increase insulin sensitivity, and improve cardiovascular health.

We, too, love cinnamon, but we realized that the most popular brand of cinnamon contains a compound called coumarin, which in large amounts is toxic to the liver. In small amounts, regular cinnamon is not harmful, but if you're like us and eat a lot of cinnamon, it's better to use Ceylon cinnamon, which we always have on our spice shelf. It's full of antioxidants for our intestinal flora!

And how did it all end for Hugo Cinnamon? Thanks for asking—he lived to be over a hundred years old.

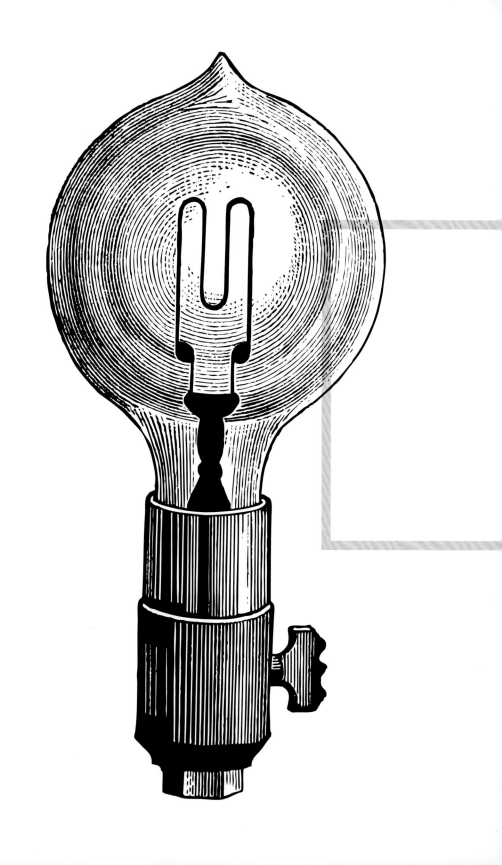

!

ONE EXTRA, SECRET, CHAPTER

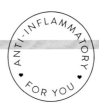

Lina and Mia are lounging on the couch, each with a laptop on her knee, arguing about whether to toss out the extra, secret chapter in the book or not.

– Wait a minute, how do you feel about the extra chapter? Maybe it won't be cool to act like a moralizing auntie.

– No, that won't be welcome. However, it's going to be tough to turn a blind eye to facts.

– Sure, a few years ago we didn't have a clue about how serious the situation actually is. Today, we're happy we had our eyes opened.

– That's so true—and this chapter adds another dimension, too. People's lifestyles don't just bring on consequences for each person, but it spills over into society as a whole.

Mia looks at Lina. Lina looks at Pyret. Pyret looks at the wall.

What the heck, let's keep it. Do you have the energy to listen some more?

We're not just interested in intestinal flora and food; we're quite into politics, too. Now that we've made it through the entire book, we know research proves that a lifestyle built on poor nutrition, little or no exercise, lots of stress, and exposure to chemicals contributes to the dramatic increase of many chronic diseases among children as well as adults. Even though no one disputes the fact that the majority of our illnesses are linked to our lifestyle and that they can be prevented to a great degree, there is a worrying silence coming from politicians. The politics of health care focuses mostly on putting out fires and pushing money toward acute needs. I'm sure we can agree that we need more nurses, but if we don't begin to treat the reason why we need more nurses, we will only keep solving acute problems. Soon, millions of dollars will be spent, and millions after that.

In our present day, we read on almost a daily basis that our health care is on its knees. What does the future hold if the prognosis is indeed showing a tripling rate of chronic illness before the year 2050 actually materializes? We can't make the math add up, and by the looks of things neither can the WHO (World Health Organization). The WHO even warns us that the cost of this huge increase in lifestyle-caused diseases will be so high that our tax-financed health care system might collapse. We live longer, but at the same time the number of chronic illnesses increases. Chronic illnesses now strike people at a much younger age, which means that more people will need many more years of care to keep their health in check. How can we solve this problem? How do we find a balance? And who really bears the biggest responsibility—the individual or society?

Society does, of course. People's health is, without a doubt, a societal problem. Food and, in the long run, our health have become class issues. This is a natural outgrowth of the food industry focusing on finding food that is cheap to manufacture. Look at what it costs to feed a family with white bread, pasta, sausage, chips, and soda for one month, and compare the amount with what it costs to feed that family organic vegetables and antioxidant-rich grains. You'll see that most people today have to eat nutrient-poor stomach fillers, and only a minority consume the recommended amount of vegetables and fiber. Why can't it be the other way around, that it is more affordable for people to eat well?

Bearing in mind that we live in Sweden, a country that uses taxes diligently as a tool, this should be relatively simple. Tax unhealthy food to make it more expensive to purchase; and instead of keeping healthy food out of reach for most people (as is the case today), remove the sales tax on health-sustaining food.

Fig. #9

WHAT DOES THIS PICTURE REPRESENT?

Breakfast order   **Room:** 121

Parent's breakfast:

Bread: White ☐   Dark ☐   Crispbread ☒

Cheese ☐   Ham ☐

Beverage: Coffee ☒   Tea ☐   Milk ☒   Sugar ☐

Juice: Apple ☐   Orange ☐

Child's breakfast:

Bread: White ☐   Dark ☒   Crispbread ☐

Cheese ☒   Ham ☐

Beverage: Apple ☒   Orange ☐ Chocolate drink ☐   Fruit yogurt ☒

Infant formula ☐

Oatmeal ☐   Puree ☐

Correct answer: A sample breakfast for a parent/patient at the Karolinska Hospital in Stockholm, Sweden

Companies that make subpar food should be given incentives to change their production over to healthy foods. It should become more profitable for manufacturers to produce a range of options that is implementable over the long haul. The banning of trans-fats in many countries proves that it's possible to legislate away harmful additives from our foods. Instead of allocating all our resources to help those who have eaten themselves into a state of poor health, shouldn't we make an effort to prevent them from eating that way in the first place, for goodness, sake?

If we take a look at what is being served in the public sector, it's obvious who's at fault.

It's time for a pop quiz.
What does the picture on page 178 show?
1 A classic Sunday breakfast
2 Our five-year-olds' breakfast wish list
3 A patient breakfast at the Karolinska Hospital in Stockholm, Sweden

Yes, we know you might be starting to find us a bit tiresome. After all, can't you catch a break from figuring out what's healthy and what's harmful, especially when you're sick? Of course you can. You really shouldn't have to think about this stuff at all. However, the hospital should give it some thought and serve food that helps heal the body and not . . . well, dammit, let's go over that list again. Chocolate drink? White bread? Fruit yogurt? Processed meat? It may not be bad for you over a short spell, but in our opinion this is hugely important because of the message it conveys. We see it everywhere—in kindergartens, schools, elder care facilities, and hospitals—nutrient-poor ingredients, lots of added sugar, pesticides, and additives, and cheap meat from countries where the use of large amounts of antibiotics in animal farming is widespread. If society's health care, academic, and welfare institutions don't even set the bar high when it comes to the nutritional value in their food, how can we expect everyone else to do it at home?

Our hearts pound hardest when we broach the topic of food in schools. Good habits start early in life, and as a result schools provide an ideal environment for teaching children healthy eating habits. Nutrient-rich food is proven to be better for students' concentration and ease of learning, and it also makes for calmer groups and classes.

Sadly, studies reveal that only a few schools have succeeded in meeting the nutritional requirement of healthy school food. Every day, approximately 30.4 million meals are served to American students in public and nonprofit private schools that are part of the National School Lunch Program (NSLP), a federally assisted meal program. These millions of meals cost the NSLP about 13.6 billion dollars a year. Billions of dollars going mostly to feed Darth Vader. What a waste.

We feel it's high time that politicians pass legislation and insist on higher standards from companies that are involved in the production of food for kindergartens, schools, hospitals, assisted living facilities, and elder care. The minimum requirement should be that food simply be nutritious and contribute to good health. Of course, it will cost a few more dollars to go from stomach fillers to nutritious food that backs Luke and his army, but when we think of the high cost of health care resulting from the consumption of bad food, we daresay you'll get your money back tenfold.

So, the correct answer to our pop quiz is of course 3) the patients' breakfast at Karolinska Hospital. Lina was handed that sheet of paper one year ago when she spent a night at the hospital with her five-year-old son. It's a good thing Carl didn't know how to read; he would have ordered the chocolate drink, fruit yogurt, and a sandwich on white bread, and in doing so would have already exceeded the RDI (recommended daily intake) of sugar per day, per child, at as early as 7:30 a.m.

Epilogue

When we were children, we used to play a game called "Fowl, fish, or in-between." The rules were very simple. Mia would ask Lina: "Fowl, fish, or in-between?" and Lina would answer: "Fowl." Mia would start to look in all the high-up places around the room until she found the loot at the top of a bookshelf. Lina and Mia laughed—very smart.

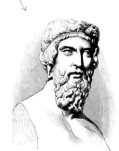

Plato, again

Today, when people ask us "Fowl, fish, or in-between?" they don't look very playful. They seem to be inquiring about what we eat. Do we eat fowl? (Absolutely!) Fish? (Yes, that too, quite often.) But what do we eat in-between? (Lots and lots of vegetables in different colors, shapes, and textures.)

As we write this, we are taking a bite of a vegetarian noodle salad with fresh cilantro, chili peppers, and cashews, along with some home-baked seed crackers. It smells so good we can hardly control ourselves. And with the scent of cilantro in our nostrils, we close our laptops for the last time and raise our glasses of filtered water, because we have finally written the final word in this book.

(This is in the ideal world, of course. In the real world we have just poured ourselves a margarita.)

REFERENCES

Baptist JA, Carvalho RC, "Indirect determination of Amadori compounds in milk-based products by HPLC/ ELSD/UV as an index of protein detorioration." [sic] *Food Res Intenat,* 2004; 37:739-47.

Bengmark S. "Advanced glycation and lipoxidation end products— amplifiers of inflammation: the role of food." *JPEN Parenter Enteral Nutr,* 2007;31(5):430-40.

Bengmark S. "Nutritional modulation of acute and 'chronic' phase response." *Nutrition,* 2001;17:489-495.

Bengmark S. "Bio-ecological Control of the Gastrointestinal Tract: The Role of Flora and Supplemented Pro-and Synbiotics." *Gastroenterol Clin North Am,* 2005;34:413-436.

Bengmark S. "Impact of nutrition on ageing and disease." *Curr Opin Nutr Metab Care,* 2006;9:2-7.

Bengmark S. "Curcumin, an atoxic antioxidant and natural NFkappaB, cyclooxygenase-2, lipooxygenase, and inducible nitric oxide synthase inhibitor: A shield against acute and chronic diseases." *JPEN J Parenter Enteral Nutr,* 2006; 30(1):45-51.

Bierhaus A, Humpert PM, Morcos M, Wendt T, Chavakis T, Arnold B, et al. "Understanding RAGE, the receptor for advanced glycation end products." *J Mol Med,* 2005;83(11):876-86.

Bohlender JM, Franke S, Stein G, Wolf G. "Advanced glycation end products and the kidney." *Am J Physiol Renal Physiol,* 2005;289(4):F645-59.

Brandtzaeg P, Halstensen TS, Krajci P, Kett K, Kvale D, Rognum TO, et al. "Immunobiology and immunopathology of human gut mucosa: Humoral immunity and intraepithelial lymphocytes." *Gastroenterology,* 1989;97(6):1562-84.

Carroll KK. "Experimental evidence of dietary factors and hormone-dependent cancers." *Cancer Res,* 1975;35(11Pt.2):3374-83.

Chainani, Wu N. "Safety and anti-inflammatory activity of curcumin: a component of turmeric (Cucurma Longa)." *J Alternative and Complementary Medicine,* 2003;9:161-168.

Clemente JC et al. "The microbiome of uncontacted Amerindians." *Science Advance,* 2015;1(3).

Colin Campbell and Thomas M Campbell, *The China Study* (Benbella Books), 2005.

Dewulf EM et al. "Gut microbiome, obesity, and metabolic dysfunction." *JCI*, Volume 121, Issue 6 2013;62:1112-1121.

Dina M, Abbate R, Gensini GF, Casini A, Sofi F. "Vegetarian, vegan diets and multiple health outcomes: a systematic review with meta-analysis of observational studies." *Crit Rev Food Sci Nutr*, published online February 6, 2016.

Fernholm A, *Det sötaste vi har* (Natur & Kultur), 2014.

Fernholm A, *Ett sötare blod* (Natur & Kultur), 2012.

Fontana L, Meyer TE, Klein S, Holloszy JO. "Long-term low-calorie low-protein vegan diet and endurance exercise are associated with low cardiometabolic risk." *Rejuvenation Res*, 2007;10(2):225-34.

Guess ND et al. *Ann Nutr Metab*, 2015:17;68:26-34.

Michael Gregor and Gene Stone, *How Not to Die* (Macmillan), 2016.

Hu FB, Manson JE, Stampfer MJ, Colditz G, Liu S, Solomon CG, et al. "Diet, lifestyle and the risk of type 2 diabetes mellitus in women." *N Engl J Med*, 2001;34511)5:790-7.

Jiang R, Paik DC, Hankinson JL, Barr RG. "Cured meat consumption, lung function, and chronic obstructive pulmonary disease among United States adults." *Am J Respir Crit Care Med,* 2007;175(8):798-804.

Jonsson D, *Magsmart* (Fitnessförlaget), 2016.

Leaf A, Weber PC. "Cardiovascular effects of n-3 fatty acids." *N Engl J Med*, 1988;318(9):549-57.

Ludvigsson J. "Why diabetes incidence increases-A unifying theory." *Ann N Y Acad Sci,* 2006;1079:374-382.

Madden JaJ, Hunter JO. "A review of the gut micro ora in irritable bowel syndrome and the effects of probiotics." *Br J Nutr,* 2002;88(suppl 1):S67-s72.

Maki KC et al. "Resistant Starch from High-Amylose Maize Increases Insulin Sensitivity in Overweight and Obese Men." *J Nutr*, 2012;142:717-723.

Malekinejad H, Scherpenisse P, Bergwerff AA. "Naturally occurring estrogens in processed milk and in raw milk (from gestated cows)." *Agric Food Chem*, 2006;54(26):9785-91.

Mattson MP. "Will caloric restriction and folate protect against AD and PD?" *Neurology*, 2003;60(4):690-5.

Meyer TE, Kovács SJ, Ehsani AA, Holloszy JO, Fontana L. "Long-term caloric restriction ameliorates the decline in diastolic function in humans." *J Am Coo Cardiol* 2006;a47(2):398-402.

Paulún F. *Sanningen om GI* (Fitnessförlaget), 2008.

Platz EA, Willett WC, Colditz GA, Rimm EB, Spiegelman D, Giovannucci E. "Proportion of colon cancer risk that might be preventable in a cohort of middle-aged US men." *Cancer Causes Control*, 2000;11.

Sebeková K, Krajcoviová-Kudlacková M, Schinzel R, Faist V, Klvanová J, Heidland A. "Plasma levels of advanced glycation end products in healthy, long-term vegetarians and subjects on a western mixed diet." *Eur J Nutr*, 2001;40(6):275-81.

Stampfer MJ, Hu FB, Manson JE, Rimm EB, Willett WC. "Primary prevention of coronary heart disease in women through diet and lifestyle." *N Engl J Med*, 2000;343(1):16-22.

Stuyven E et al. "Oral administration of beta-1,3/1,6-glucan Macrogard fails to enhance the mucosal immune response following oral F4 fimbrial immunisation in gnotobiotic pigs." *Vet Immunol Immunopathol*, 2009;128:60-66.

Talbott SM, Talbott JA. "Baker's yeast beta-glucan supplement reduces upper respiratory symptoms and improves mood state in stressed women." *J AmColl Nutr*, 2012;31:295-300.

Tlaskalova-Hogenova H, Tuckova L, Stepankova R, Hudcovic T, Palova-Jelinkova L, Kozakova H. "Involvement of innate immunity in the development of in amatory [sic] and autoimmune diseases." *Ann N Y Acad Sci*, 2005 Jun;1051:787-798.

Vetvicka V, Vetvickova J. "Glucan Supplementation Has Strong Anti-melanoma Effects: Role of NK Cells." *Anticancer Res*, 2015;35:5287-5292.

Wolever TNS, Jenkins DJA. "Effect of dietary fiber and foods on carbohydrate metabolism. In GA Spiller, editor." *Handbook of Dietary Fiber in Human Nutrition*, CRC Press, Boca Raton, FL, 1993;111-152.

OUR THANKS GO TO

Stig & Marianne Bengmark
Anna Lindelöw
Cecilia Viklund
Linnéa von Zweigbergk
Ulrika Ekblom
Team Hawaii
Marie Sandahl
Plato
Ann Fernholm
David Stenholz
Fredrik Paulún
George Lucas
Benicio del Toro

Nybrogatan 38
Emil
The four small hooligans—Carl, Juni,
Ludde, and Ninni
Dad Jan
Mom Ann
Runken
Pyret
All other family members and friends
All blog readers—without you there
would be no book

If you miss us, you can always find us
at www.foodpharmacy.blog.

Copyright © Mia Clase and Lina Nertby Aurell
English translation © 2017 Skyhorse Publishing

First published by Bonnier Fakta, Stockholm, Sweden

All rights reserved. No part of this book may be reproduced in any manner without the express written consent of the publisher, except in the case of brief excerpts in critical reviews or articles. All inquiries should be addressed to Skyhorse Publishing, 307 West 36th Street, 11th Floor, New York, NY 10018.

Skyhorse Publishing books may be purchased in bulk at special discounts for sales promotion, corporate gifts, fund-raising, or educational purposes. Special editions can also be created to specifications. For details, contact the Special Sales Department, Skyhorse Publishing, 307 West 36th Street, 11th Floor, New York, NY 10018 or info@skyhorsepublishing.com.

Skyhorse® and Skyhorse Publishing® are registered trademarks of Skyhorse Publishing, Inc.®, a Delaware corporation.

Visit our website at www.skyhorsepublishing.com.

10 9 8 7 6 5 4 3 2 1

Library of Congress Cataloging-in-Publication Data is available on file.

Photo: Ulrika Ekblom
Design: Anna Lindelöv
Illustration page 3 and collage on end papers ©Wellcome Images, wellcomeimages.org
Illustration pages 5 and 24 © Marie Sandahl
Illustrations pages 8, 11, 32, 48, 88, 105, 136, 149, 160, 166, 174, 181 © Shutterstock
Picture page 18 © Team Hawaii

Print ISBN: 978-1-5107-2348-1
Ebook ISBN: 978-1-5107-2351-1

Printed in China

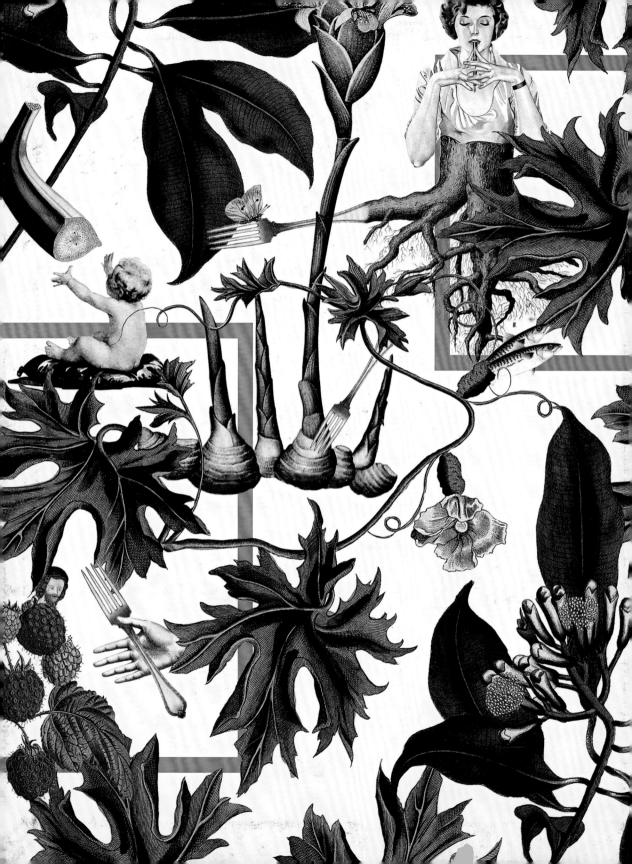